*Im*perfectly natural home

Imperfectly natural home

Everything you need to know to create a healthy, natural home

Janey Lee Grace

First published in Great Britain in 2008 by
Orion Books
an imprint of the Orion Publishing Group Ltd
Orion House, 5 Upper St Martin's Lane,
London WC2H 9EA
An Hachette Livre UK Company

1 3 5 7 9 10 8 6 4 2

A CIP catalogue record for this book is available
from the British Library.

ISBN: 978 0 7528 8582 7

Designed by Goldust Design
Printed in Spain by Cayfosa Quebecor

The Orion Publishing Group's policy is to use papers that are natural, renewable and recyclable and
made from wood grown in sustainable forests. The logging and manufacturing processes are expected
to conform to the environmental regulations of the country of origin.

www.orionbooks.co.uk

Acknowledgements

Thanks to everyone at Orion books. Euan Thorneycroft at AM Heath and Tony Fitzpatrick at People Matter TV. Thanks also to Fiona Robson and Gabrielle Packer for their admin support (and endless supplies of imperfectly natural mugs of tea).

Thanks again to Steve Wright and Tim Smith at Radio 2, who have endured another year musing over my wacky 'holistic' ideals.

Currently making my own very imperfectly natural (but healthy) home an unholy mess are my four gorgeous kids, Sonny, Buddy, Rocky and Lulu, who constantly amaze me with their undying devotion to emptying the compost crock (!) and much love and thanks to Simon, without whom I couldn't have managed any of this.

Finally thanks to all the natural/eco companies who have introduced me to so many innovative natural/eco products, to my wonderful virtual friends on my forum at **www.imperfectlynatural.com** and to Nikki and Sarah, the Imperfectly Natural 'mod-fairies'.

Contents

6 Household appliances

7 Natural remedies

8 Personal Care

9 Children

10 Clothing, furnishings and fabrics

11 Organising and clutter-clearing

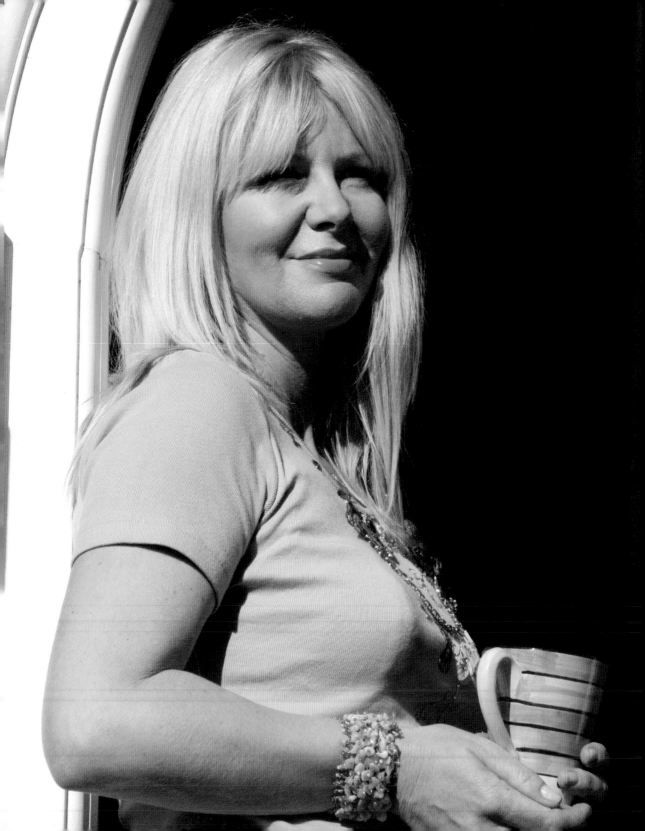

Introduction

Most of us are well aware of the basics of being eco-friendly, but I wonder if it all just seems like yet another chore? If you're only really rather reluctantly making minimal changes in order to avoid the rubbish police fining you for slipping a bit of plastic into your cardboard recycling container, then you won't be alone. Trying to be an eco warrior can be exhausting, and quite honestly, with all the extra stress, our relationships will break down quicker than compost if we don't get to grips with a workable way of being 'green' and 'holistic' – albeit imperfectly.

The mantra that has got me out of many an accusation of being a hypocrite is that I am 'imperfect'. Yes, I care about the environment; I want to leave some of the earth's resources around for my four children and their children. And I care about my health too, as we all do. Of course many people believe that the health service will take care of that, but I'm not prepared to automatically trust that the right pill or surgical procedure will be administered just when I require it, and I don't want to spend hours queuing up to get a sick note to take time off work: I want to be well. I believe we should take back control and look at prevention rather than cure, holistically – by which I mean across the whole spectrum. I'm only human and, like all of us, busy, and I don't do anything like as much as I should to care for my own health or that of the planet: I am still, if truth be told, only a shade on from lime green.

> *'Be grateful for the home you have, knowing that at this moment all you have is all you need.'*
> Sarah Ban, Breathnatch

But what I lack in depth of hue I hope I make up for in my enthusiasm for a simpler, healthier existence, though for me I confess much of it began for selfish reasons for my own health and well-being. In this book I hope to be able to pass some of that on to you – the enthusiasm, not the selfishness!

I won't badger or harass you, and I'm definitely not trying to make you feel guilty for the bits you're not doing. I'll help you rejoice and celebrate the fact that by making the first small change, you can make a big difference. Interestingly if you start with your own health and well-being, you often find that you can tick the 'green' box in the process.

Like me you're probably way too busy to live a totally sustainable self-sufficient existence. While I appreciate the whole concept of 'slowing down', the reality is that some days I can't catch my own tail as I rocket through my daily chores at 100 miles an hour, and juggle four kids and career, so I simply can't just 'chill'. The good news, though, is that I think we can have our eco/natural cake and eat it. I think it's okay to start small and build on good intentions, and if through this book I can point you in the direction of just one ethical, natural, fairly traded alternative that will help your health and in the process help save the environment, then I'll be a very happy little Kermit (he's very green, if you're too young to remember the Muppets).

I'll skim over what you may consider the ultimate dream, a purpose-built eco home, to the reality that is the average home, whether for you that means a suburban semi, a room in a shared house, an old rambling family cottage, a barge or bedsit. Whatever your dwelling, you can make your home environment as natural as possible. That doesn't mean I'm suggesting we all build log cabins and burn incense sticks: this is a concept that works across all styles, tastes and budgets. And you can do this not just for the sake of being worthy but to really make a difference to your own personal health and well-being, and in doing so you'll hopefully do your bit towards energy saving and the green cause too.

I will fast-track you to the best products, services and ideas to get you started. Some will cost you next to nothing, so you'll save cash too. Many of my tips are 'old style' and you'll wonder why you didn't ditch your synthetic chemical cleaning products years ago and dig out the lemons, bicarbonate of soda and elbow grease.

I'll look at your home and suggest ways to improve its 'holistic health'. I'll cover energy and water saving, and look at interiors, with a particular emphasis on how colours, textures and textiles affect our moods and well-being. I'll touch on the more common-sense bits of feng shui and how you can apply it to enhance your life. I'll explore the best eco furnishings and appliances and inspire you to 'reduce, re-use and recycle'. I'm not an experienced builder, maintenance gal or interior designer (sadly), so I won't get too technical over anything, but I will point you in the direction of the best books and websites so that you can do your own research. This is a still relatively new but fast-growing industry – fairly traded natural products, sustainable materials, energy-saving gadgets and eco building supplies have never been more in abundance – and I'll help you to sort the passionate ethical ones from the 'jump on the green bandwagon' charlatans.

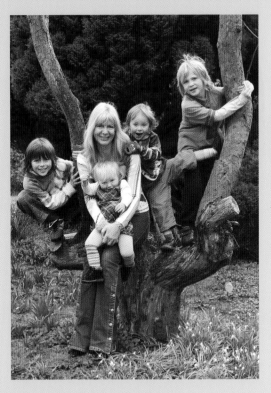

I'll also, perhaps surprisingly, include a chapter about Christmas. I know it comes but once a year, but for many of us how we celebrate it is pivotal to our perception of a happy, balanced home. It's often the busiest time of the year and the time when we spend the most money and use the most resources, but there are ways to reduce, re-use and recycle and still have a fantastic Christmas.

If at any point you start feeling inadequate and thinking you'll never make that lovely shade of olive, just move to another section of the book. We're all at a different stage of our imperfectly natural 'journey' and life is too short to be beating yourself up about the wine bottle you didn't recycle or the disposable nappy you've just chucked away. It's okay to make some imperfect compromises, but we all know small changes can make a big difference, so together we'll sow the seeds of organic living that contribute to healthy homes and lives.

'Home is any four walls that enclose the right person.'
Helen Rowland, American journalist

YOUR HOME AND HOW IT AFFECTS YOUR WELL-BEING

We spend 65 per cent of our lives at home. Most of us feel that our home is our castle and a safe haven from the outside world. I wish it were so, and trust me I don't want to harass and scaremonger you into feeling you need to move house, but we should be aware of some of the potential problems and health hazards that are associated with modern living. There are many eco warriors around right now, including some government officials who will be coercing us and even taxing us into making changes for the good of the planet, and that's all fine, but I'd present this slightly differently, and say let's look at how our personal environment, our living space or the way we live is affecting our health and well-being. Once we're aware, we as individuals can make a few often very simple changes and the great news is that there are so many alternatives now available it is possible to counter some of the hazards.

'Home – that blessed word, which opens to the human heart the most perfect glimpse of Heaven, and helps to carry it thither, as on an angel's wings.'

Lydia M. Child, writer, abolitionist

Back in the Second World War, food rationing and scarcity meant that people ate a healthy, balanced diet. Undoubtedly they ate smaller amounts of food with less fat, sugar and dairy products, and adequate but fairly small amounts of protein in the form of meat and fish. Importantly, they ate lots more vegetables, particularly with the highly successful 'Dig for Victory' campaign, which encouraged everyone with a garden to transform it into a mini allotment – it's estimated that over 1.4 million people had their own allotment. They also ate seasonal organic food. Strawberries in winter weren't an option, and the fresh fruit and vegetables often grown in their own gardens was organic because they simply didn't have pesticides available. It is thought that the average calorie intake was reduced from over 3,000 to approximately 2,800 calories a day.

People were naturally 'greener' in terms of energy consumption too. Houses were mostly draughty and cold rather than the artificially 'heated and sealed' units most of us live in now. I can clearly remember the council house

I grew up in as a child. We had no central heating and in the winter shivering upstairs to the freezing cold loo was excruciating, but it's probably the reason that I can now easily tolerate the cold, and I'm usually the one telling all my family who huddle around the radiators to stop being 'nesh' (that's a northern saying for feeling the cold easily).

But we're now in the age of convenience, comfort and all mod cons, and a frightening amount of suspect new materials are used in building and furnishing our homes. Far from being a safe haven from the polluted outside world our homes, offices and places of work actually contain more pollution than the average street corner or busy roadside.

In the excellent book *Your Healthy Home*, a 'What Doctors Don't Tell You' publication edited by Lynne McTaggart, the authors looked at a long-term study of people living in three different types of areas in the United States: one group in a highly industrialised area, one in a semi-industrialised area and one group in a rural area. By means of an automatic pump attached to their chests they sampled the air of over 350 people as they went about their daily lives and work. The results were striking. They found that in a typical day at work and home these people breathed in more hazardous chemicals when they were indoors than when they were in their own gardens. In semi-industrialised and even rural areas, the levels of air chemicals were between five and ten times higher indoors than outside.

Because of the low-level exposure to synthetic potentially toxic chemicals found in our carpets, walls, furniture and furnishings we are more prone to symptoms such as headaches, insomnia, fatigue and allergies, and most of us just think that is normal. Interestingly when you do something to reduce the pollutants around your home you often feel an increased energy and sense of well-being.

But what are the indoor air pollutants? Well, we've all heard about volatile organic compounds (VOCs) – yet the word 'organic' has become something to aspire to in our foods, skincare and clothing, so aren't they okay? Well, no. They're derived from petrochemicals and at room temperature they release vapours. They're in just about everything, sadly, including plywood, carpets, synthetic fabrics and furnishings, normal household paint and even cleaning products.

We all know that awful chemical whiff when a room has just been painted. Both oil-based and water-based paints contain benzene, which is a known human carcinogen. Then there's the lead in house paint. I am fearful that my very old house, which is rented, could have more than the supposedly safe level of two per cent lead carbonate or lead sulphate. In Europe some exterior paints still contain lead, even though it's been banned in America.

I remember that when I ordered a new sofa a few years back, the supplier offered me a protective 'sealant' – a sort of stain-resistant coating to keep it clean for longer (in fact I think it came with a ten-year guarantee). I'm too scared to think what that contained! I refused it, so yes, a few years on I have a rather grubby couch, but perhaps we're all healthier for it.

It's not just furnishings, though. Not long ago, I bought a suitcase from a high-street store. It was sealed in plastic. Why, oh why, would a bag need to be within a bag? Well, possibly to stop the smell. When I unsealed it I nearly keeled over from the fumes of the formaldehyde, which I assume had been released from the synthetic fabric or adhesives used.

Then we have to be concerned about the pesticides in our homes. Not just the insecticides that are sprayed so liberally to control woodworm; many of us also spray our carpets, and even our clothes, with insecticides to keep away moths, and of course if we come into the house wearing our outdoor shoes we'll walk a lot of unnecessary dirt and possibly more pesticides over our carpeted areas. Add to this the effects of dust mites and moulds in our homes and we can start to feel very itchy and uncomfortable, as they're known triggers that can irritate the nasal passages and airways and so contribute to the rise in asthma and respiratory illnesses. Fortunately we can reduce our exposure to pesticides and other chemicals in foods by eating locally sourced organic fruit and veg and drinking filtered water, and if we need to ward off insects and moths there are much more natural repellents widely available.

Then we should consider the electromagnetic fields in our home. Most of us are aware that living close to power cables will probably mean you won't be offered a mortgage because of the adverse effects, but of course the jury is still out on mobile phone masts and wi-fi.

Add to that the huge amount of electrical equipment we now have in our homes compared to my childhood home and even fewer in the wartime home. Most of our 'mod cons' and gadgets are a drain on valuable energy resources and contribute to electro pollution which can result in stress, headaches and other illnesses. We can't all become 'powerless' but we can switch off our appliances when not in use, and remove all unnecessary electrical equipment, at least from the area where we sleep.

Cleaning and laundry products are a considerable proportion of the average person's weekly shopping bill and this is one area where it's easy to save money, your health and as a by-product the environment too, by replacing your cleaning products with natural alternatives.

When it comes to personal care – well, I've written about this in great detail in *Imperfectly Natural Woman* and *Imperfectly Natural Baby and Toddler*. The excellent news is that there is now a synthetic chemical-free alternative to almost everything you could wish to use, from nail varnish to baby-wipes.

> *'We shape our dwellings, and afterwards our dwellings shape us.'*
> Winston Churchill

Of course I'm not saying that any one carpet, any one bottle of detergent or even your microwave oven is going to make you ill, but I do believe that the accumulative effect of the masses of potentially toxic synthetic chemicals and pollutants that exist in our homes probably will over time, so let's address the issues now and in the process do our bit for saving the planet. I will be covering all of them in the following pages. Above all, remember I am imperfect and I'm guessing you are too, so start with something that seems fairly easy to achieve and make any other changes from there; with the bits that just seem too daunting, well, just move on. It's the 80/20 principle that's important: if you can make a start by reducing everyday synthetic chemicals and pollutants by 80 per cent, you'll be doing great, and feel better for it.

THE PERSONAL TOUCH

It's hard to describe what makes individual style so emotive. It's definitely not as simple as throwing money at it; in fact often the opposite is true – the most sparsely furnished cottage can be a delight. But ultimately whether you live in a hovel or a castle, at some point you'll find yourself emotionally attached to it.

We're inundated by magazines showing us images of beautiful houses and gardens, modern designs and traditional cosy homes, but although we may aspire to them and feel wistful that we don't own them, in reality the reason your dwelling place can be called home is because of your individual touches. These are usually simple things: a bunch of fresh lavender on a whitewashed reclaimed wood dresser, some hand-picked shells and smooth pebbles in a small wicker basket for both a visual and tactile experience. *The World of Rosamunde Pilcher* is the most gorgeous book, full of homely photographs and extracts from her poetic books set in Cornwall and Scotland. She writes about buying a new home that needed some renovation and how she felt when she finally got someone to cut the overgrown grass and prune the shrubs. Then she gets to the real issue, the washing line:

And then at the very top of the garden he set up a washing line for me, strong between three sturdy posts.
The sight of this homely contraption, viewed from my kitchen window, filled me with satisfaction. And on a bright spring morning I used it for the first time, unloading the washing machine into a wicker basket, and making my way downstairs and out into the garden. It was cold, but the first daffodils were beginning to push up through the rough grass, there was the smell of flowering currant and newly turned earth and somewhere somebody had lighted a bonfire.

What a wonderful paragraph! She expresses so well that feeling of hanging out your washing or even hanging it up to dry in your own kitchen, your own personal space where you choose which plate hangs on the wall and whether the kitchen clock will tick or chime. There is and always has been something old fashioned about the word 'home'. It's comforting and secure, safe and warm – and it's all about those personal touches.

I remember when I first left my parents' home and rented a room in a hall of residence at university. It was a small, very basic, square room with a sink and a window, but I was thrilled that, for a while at least, it was mine.

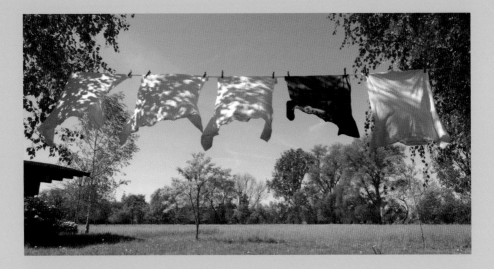

I bought posters, wall coverings, and a cheap funky bright rug and I hung beaded mobiles from the ceiling.

Even if you're in a tiny rented bed-sit, with some imagination and flair you can create a personalised home for very little cost. Brightly coloured fabrics used as throws, cushions and bunches of lavender are just one style. You might opt for an altogether more unusual arty approach and fashion a shiny wall hanging from no-longer-wanted CDs or do something artistic with bamboo. It's lovely to use natural or reclaimed materials and make a place your own. A great way to use your old photographs is to make a collage and change it around regularly, providing literally a wonderful snapshot of your life for visitors, and to remind you of friends and family.

Make sure your home in some way reflects who you are; make sure it enhances your life. Balance is what we all need to achieve and we must find that in all areas of our lives, including our relaxation as well as our work.

'Home is a name, a word, it is a strong one; stronger than magician ever spoke, or spirit ever answered to, in the strongest conjuration.' Charles Dickens

1 Cleaning

Since I wrote my first book and launched my website **www.imperfectlynatural.com**, I've been thrilled to note the huge rise in demand for natural cleaning products. I am glowing with pride (I told you I don't get out much) that I have helped to introduce the nation to balls and nuts (if you're not in the loop yet, you will be after reading the laundry section in this chapter).

Let's start with cleaning the house, though, that never-ending chore that in my house gives such satisfaction for about five minutes till the kids unwittingly trash it again. You remember the old saying 'Eat a peck of dirt . . .'? Well, it seems that there's some truth in it: being super clinically clean is not a great idea and children are much better off if allowed to rummage in the muck occasionally. Don't reel in horror. I'm not suggesting you become slovenly, but you do need to know what's in that expensive bottle of cleaning fluid that you're whooshing around, and the other 15 different bottles under your sink.

It must be stressed that all chemicals have been subject to strict testing, but being cynical I'm afraid I just don't accept that they're entirely safe for us (particularly for those whose immune systems are already compromised by allergies or respiratory problems) or kind to the environment.

Most household cleaning products contain the VCOs I mentioned earlier ('volatile organic compounds'). Sadly these compounds evaporate easily and build up in the air, so it's easy to see why studies have shown that they will aggravate asthmatics, particularly in buildings with poor ventilation. Most washing detergents have added phosphates, which will improve their cleaning power but will not be a bag of laughs for our sensitive skins. Many synthetic chemical cleaning and laundry products are manufactured from petro-chemicals, many of which are classed as hazardous waste.

They usually contain sodium laureth sulphate too, a popular foaming agent. Many of us are aware that it's best to avoid this in our skincare products, as it can cause eye irritation and dry out the skin, but we forget that it will affect us if we come into contact with it regularly while washing up and cleaning the house. Many products also contain formaldehyde, propellants (often used as pressurised sprays), lauramine oxide (another skin irritant) alcohol and synthetic fragrances, which can trigger asthma attacks, and can even be hormone-disrupting. Many

> *'Housework is what a woman does that nobody notices unless she hasn't done it.'*
>
> Evan Esar, American humorist

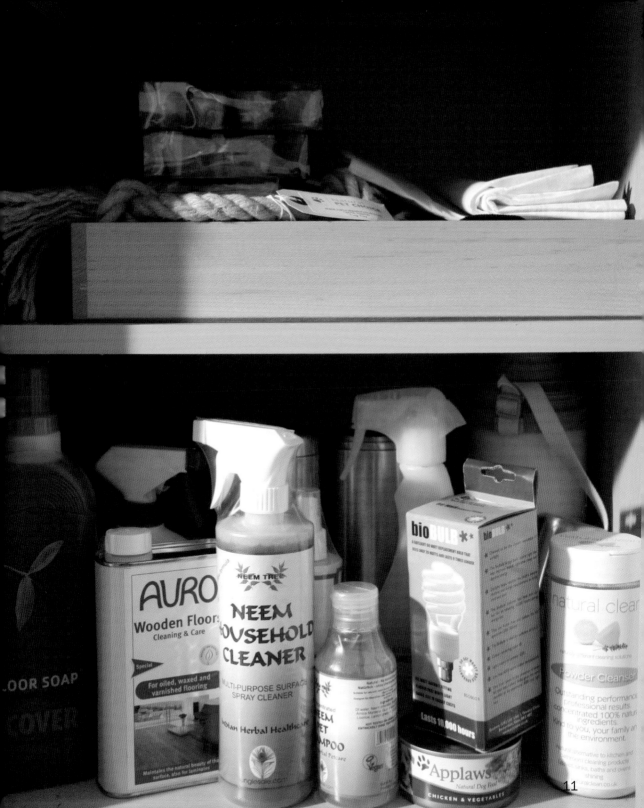

people believe that the cocktail of such synthetic chemicals contributes to allergies in children. Everything has to be cleaned, or else we'll all get ill, but then again it seems that if we continue to use chemical cleaners we'll get ill anyway.

So household cleaning products and air fresheners, particularly those which contain 'parfum' or fragrance which can contain hormone-disrupting artificial musks, could give us headaches, increase symptoms of asthma and worse, but what do they do to the environment?

Well, most commercial cleaning products don't biodegrade, or they take ages, possibly years, to break down. Phosphates are powerful fertilisers and can stimulate the growth of algae, using up oxygen in the water potentially killing the fish; then the chemicals are making their way into the 'food chain' and so it goes on. Artificial musks and perfumes used to give aroma to products build up in waterways and can harm aquatic life.

I could go on and scare you with a whole host of other chemical names, but perhaps it's better to take the optimistic approach. The good news is that there are many alternatives available now that are kinder to us and to the environment. We need to look for the ones that biodegrade easily, and are plant or vegetable based, using essential oils if fragrance is needed, and containing no artificial perfume (which can be chronically irritating to anyone with sensitive skin and breathing problems) or colorants (known carcinogens which are entirely useless). And just because a detergent is 'green' in colour it won't make it clean any more effectively.

So what are the alternatives? Thankfully there are lots, from companies using kinder plant-based chemicals to going back 50 years and getting out the lemon juice, vinegar and a large dollop of elbow grease. Let's start with the eco-friendly commercial options before we get to the 'make your own'.

GREEN CLEANING PRODUCTS

Ecover are the leaders in the field and I have a huge amount of time for this company dedicated to sustainability as well as health and ecological causes. Their first factory near Antwerp is a totally eco-friendly green building with a 5,000 square metre green roof – literally a meadow of vegetation. The management team use eco-friendly cars and the staff are rewarded for cycling or using car share schemes. It is arguably the world's most ecological factory. They are the one big company who have managed to jostle alongside Procter and Gamble and Unilever in the supermarkets and consequently they are the best known. Their loo cleaner is fantastic, as is their integrated washing powder and laundry bleach. Oh, and I love the little slogan on their washing up liquid: 'Does the dishes not the fishes'! Their packaging is recyclable or refillable and you can buy in bulk from www.ecotopia.co.uk.

Though Ecover claim about 90 per cent of the UK's green cleaning sales, they now have some serious competition from UK-based companies such as Bio D (www.biode gradable.biz), who do what they say on the tin – their main focus is on biodegradability. Clearspring (www.faithinnature.co.uk) is another excellent UK company who have an excellent range of detergents.

Both brands are available in good health food shops and from www.greenshop.co.uk.

Marks & Spencer have got in on the act with Naturally Inspired, their range of eco-cleaners. I found the bathroom cleaner quite effective, with a reasonable fruity kind of smell. There's also John Lewis now offering Method, which works well. They claim their products are biodegradable but they do use some synthetic chemicals to increase their efficiency; couple that with the fact that some of the products are flown in from the United States and you wonder how environmentally friendly they really are.

Then there's the little'uns, including companies like Natural Clean (www.naturalclean.co.uk), set up by a couple of mums who quite frankly thought they could do better for their children's skin and environment, so they developed their own range of excellent cleaning products, such as the best Orange Degreaser ever.

One of my favourite all-purpose cleaners is called Budge, from another UK company, Living Clean (www.livingclean.co.uk).

The very ethical company Daylesford (www.daylesfordorganic.com), who make great organic foods, now do natural cleaning products, including an excellent loo cleaner with rosemary.

Because we've all become accustomed over the years to that lovely fresh pine smell or that chemical lemon whiff, some people really don't think their bathroom or their washing is clean unless it smells of CIF or Comfort respectively. To this end enter into the realm of the wondrous Home Scents (www.homescents.co.uk), a company who absolutely realise that we want easy-to-use cleaning products and a few fragrant finishing touches too. Their products are handmade using 100 per cent pure essential oils.

Their room sprays are fantastic – if you choose not to follow my advice and make your own (see page 18) – and their Ironing Water is gorgeous: trust me, it's not often I get the iron out, but it was a case of needs must last week with a linen skirt so I thought I'd try it, and now I'm hooked – gorgeous light fragrance, luxury really.

Then there's the excellent company Junglesale (www.junglesale.com) who sell pure neem products. The lovely guy who runs Junglesale was exhibiting his neem-based products at a health fair and a customer said to him, 'I find it hard to believe that your household cleaner is as natural as you make out. Surely there are some synthetic chemicals in it?' Before her eyes he proceeded to take a swig directly from the bottle to prove it contained nothing scary whatsoever. The client placed a large order! That's how safe our cleaning products should be!

When buying cleaning products, opt for ones that claim they are non-toxic and are made with plant and natural mineral ingredients, with no phosphates, chlorine or optical brighteners. Also look for ones that say

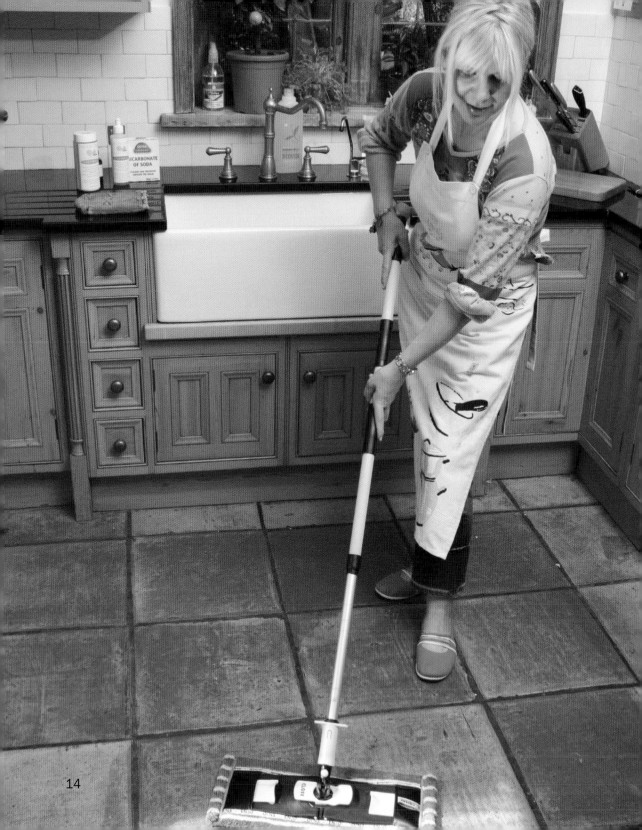

'not tested on animals' and do not contain 'parfum' or any synthetic fragrances.

It's also good to look for products that state that they are biodegradable and come in recyclable packaging. Some of my favourite ethical companies for household cleaning products are:

www.naturalclean.co.uk
www.livingclean.co.uk
www.perledeprovence.co.uk
www.biodegradable.biz
www.clearspring.co.uk
www.natural-house.co.uk
www.lemonburst.co.uk

CLEANING TOOLS

Oh, the joys of microfibre cloths, available now in your regular £1 shop! I bought the original and best 'e-cloth' and it's brilliant. It's a general-purpose cloth made of millions of tiny fibres that will absorb the grease and the dirt. You can use it dry to polish furniture but mostly I use it with a drop of tea tree oil and nothing else to clean surfaces, the loo, bath, whatever. They reckon it can be washed up to 300 times and it requires no cleaning product. Seems incredible, doesn't it? I now make sure I've got lots of them and use them for just about everything. They cost about £4.99 for two from www.e-cloth.com.

I like Enjo (www.enjo.net) products too. The company has several distributors who may put you off with their zealous passion (it's not normal to be that thrilled about cleaning, is it?) but there's no doubt their range is unique. I use their 'mitt', made from super-absorbent microfibres, and a pretty cool telescopic mop (pictured), which cleans a really dirty kitchen floor with just water. I don't know how but it works. After years of throwing out hopeless mops I feel quite liberated (see, it is getting to me, I admit it – I'm going bonkers!).

You can also get a 'universal cleaning block', which is an ingenious way of cleaning without chemicals. It's basically a tough foam block with an abrasive effect that can be run under water and then rubbed against metal, wood, glass and ceramics. It's only about £2.95 from www.naturalcollection.com.

If you have access to a steam cleaner – you can pick them up for about £50, possibly less, or on Freecycle, (see page 53) – you've got an instant quick way to clean just about all surfaces, walls, furniture, even carpets. Obviously the steam loosens the dirt, though, so you'll need to mop it up afterwards. A small one is fine so long as you're happy to keep refilling it with water. If you're doing a serious spring clean, consider hiring an industrial one for the day or ask around your neighbours to see if they've one you can borrow.

GOING OLD STYLE

But what about the old-style, back-to-the-fifties cleaning methods? Well, they so appeal to me, not because I'm a sucker for punishment and I want to be on my hands and knees like a 1950s housewife scrubbing floors, but because there's something intrinsically satisfying about cleaning your windows with vinegar and

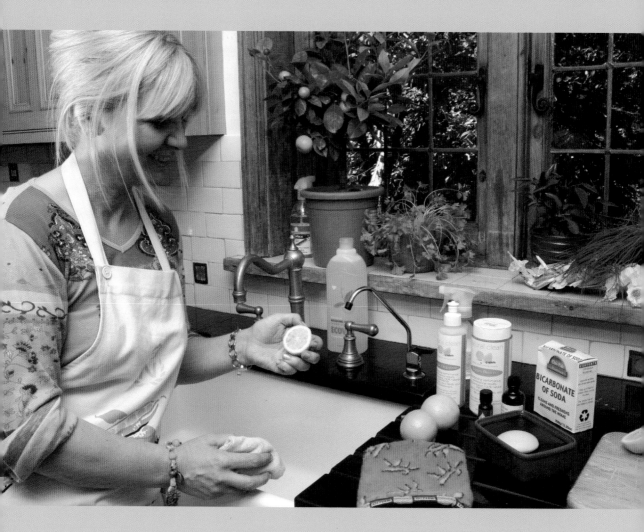

newspaper and your kitchen sink with what's left over of the lemon that you made your salad dressing from. You know not only that your house is clean – naturally clean – but also that you and you kids are healthy, not intoxicated by a chemical mix, and that you are not contributing to further destruction of the precious planet.

A couple of years ago we had an au pair girl from Romania. She was fantastic and became a dear friend, godmother to my baby and all-round 'angel'. Before she arrived, she told me in her emails that she 'loved cleaning' (I resisted from asking 'Pardon – are you nuts?' and just thought, 'Thank you, God') and sure enough, the first day she got stuck in to my messy house she donned her rubber gloves and then set about finding what she needed under the sink. But I'll never forget what happened next. I made the mistake of going out and when I got back the whole house reeked of bleach. She had looked at my collection of bicarbonate of soda, an e-cloth, a few bottles of tea tree oil and some soapnuts, and decided we must have run out of cleaning equipment. So she had taken herself off to buy bleach and all manner of synthetic chemical-laden cleaning kit. I kid you not: when I first walked through the door, I thought I'd entered a swimming pool – it's incredible how, when you're not used to it, the whiff of chlorine can hit you at 30 feet.

She came round after a while, though, and certainly she'll never throw a lemon away again. Even the mankiest oldest bit of old citrus fruit will get a rubbing round the sink in my place before it's composted.

It's worth stocking up on some natural store cupboard basics for making your own household cleaners.

Essential oils *Tea tree oil* You can buy large bottles from **www.essentiallyoils.com**. *Lemon, peppermint, lavender* You may also want to stock up on lemon or peppermint oil, plus lavender oil – depending on your choice of fragrance. Choose pure oil, not a blend.

Bicarbonate of soda I now buy it in bulk. I've used it since my student days to soak up smells, even after decorating. You can get it in most chemists or from **www.dri-pak.co.uk**. Make it into a paste with water and you can use it to clean most surfaces, polish chrome and even as a natural toothpaste (see page 86 [Personal care]).

Lemons and grapefruit Hang on to lemons till they really are spent. The last dregs of a lemon can be rubbed over a chopping board and will make any ceramic surface sparkle. Similarly, a used grapefruit makes a good 'scrubbing mitt', if you add some salt to really attack the grime (see below). Even when a lemon is thoroughly used up you can pop the skin into the cutlery drawer of the dishwasher to add a bit of extra sparkle

Salt Regular table salt makes a great abrasive scouring powder if needed.

White distilled vinegar Has many uses, from descaling kettles to cleaning loos. Buy it from any supermarket.

Citric acid You'll need this to make your own dishwasher detergent. You can find it in most pharmacies. Mix about a quarter of a cup with a quarter of a cup of household salt, one cup of bicarbonate of soda and one cup of borax; then add a little water so that it's gloopy but not runny, and about five to ten drops of eucalyptus or lemon oil. Store it in a sealed container. You'll need about two tablespoons. As well as popping lemon rind in the cutlery tray to give everything a sparkle, always use white distilled vinegar as a rinse aid. You can also use soapnut liquid (see page 24) for the dishwasher.

Borax This is good to have on hand (see page 27 [Laundry]). Many branches of high street chemists stock it now.

SMELL-BUSTING

Most standard air fresheners contain environmentally harmful CFCs and all manner of chemicals said to increase respiratory problems and headaches. It's ridiculously easy to go another route. For starters, open a window, and neutralise any smells such as paint or cigarette smoke by leaving a little bowl or carton containing bicarbonate of soda around. It's great at neutralising odours.

If you like to 'spritz', buy a plant spray and fill it with water and a couple of drops of essential oil – that's it! Too simple? Yes. If you like a fresh antiseptic kind of whiff, use tea tree oil – it's antibacterial and anti-

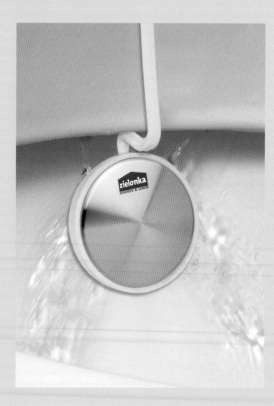

inflammatory; or you can use citronella for a lemony zing or lavender for a relaxing spritz. Most health shops carry a selection or buy from **www.essentiallyoils.com**. Sometimes it feels nice just to walk around spraying, so do that to your heart's content without damaging your nasal passages with chemicals or the ozone layer with the CFCs from an aerosol can.

The excellent 'ask the expert' section on **www.livingclean.co.uk** advises for a simple air freshener: 'Put one part white vinegar to three parts water in a plant spray with two drops of peppermint oil added.' Mmm ... I'm off to try that one ...

Natural Collection (**www.natural collection.com**) have a great range of 'smell-busters' made from high-grade stainless steel, which is said to neutralise odours as soon as it comes into contact with water or odour. Trust me, I'm no scientist and I can't in truth tell you how this works, but I have the toilet smell killer (a small stainless steel disk about five cm in diameter) hanging in my toilet bowl and I can assure you that it works. Should last longer than me, too.

There's also a stainless-steel Universal Smell Killer, and 'smell-busters' for the fridge and dishwasher, and a Shoe Smell Killer, (all from **www.vitalia-health.co.uk**) although I sometimes wonder, How do they know?

You can also get a great range of air fresheners and room sprays to suit your mood, including an amazingly zingy bathroom spray from Spiezia Organics (**www.spiezia organics.co.uk**) and a lovely relaxing one from Neal's Yard (**www.nealsyardremedies.co.uk**).

HOW TO CLEAN...

Loos I know what you're shouting: but what do you actually get down the loo with when it's really stained? Well, I can't pretend that's an easy one. I find the whole idea of loo brushes faintly disgusting – like when are they ever cleaned? For regular cleaning I use any of the excellent eco loo cleaners. I put on some rubber gloves, look the other way and get down there with a scrubbing brush followed by my toilet-dedicated Enjo cleaning mitt and some tea tree oil. When I come up for air at least the room smells 'clean' with the antiseptic whiff of the tea tree.

Then all I need to address is any extensive staining around the pan – oh God, what a horrible topic! I use the 'leave in' powder cleanser from Natural Clean (**www.naturalclean.co.uk**). Try and leave it in overnight without flushing. I've heard of pouring Coca-Cola down the loo to clear the stains from the pan, but I must admit it hasn't really worked for me. Dental tablets (designed for false teeth) are also meant to clear stains and they do seem to work better, but God knows what's in those! (Hardly chemical free or environmentally friendly, I fear.) You can make your own 'fizzing solution' with two tablespoons each of citric acid and bicarbonate of soda, or make a simple loo cleaner with plant-based washing-up liquid mixed with bicarbonate of soda, water and white vinegar. But it's elbow grease and regular cleaning that are the key.

You can also use a cup of household borax, brush it around and leave it overnight. True loo cleaning purists may recommend that if the bowl is very stained you need to remove some of the water before you get down there with the brush. In that case I can only suggest a narrow jug and a hearty spirit!

For more commercial options, there's Ecover and Bio D (see page 12), and you can also buy chlorine-free toilet bleach. Heather's oxygen bleach cleanser is based on simple minerals and naturally derived biodegradable surfactants. They say it's safer for rivers, streams and septic tank systems too. You can get it fragrance free or fragranced with orange, citrus or tea tree. Works out expensive, though, at around £5.00 for 400g from **www.kinetic4health.co.uk**.

For the loo seat I always use neat tea tree oil and wipe with an e-cloth, which goes straight into the washing machine (even imperfect old me is a bit fanatical where toilets and germ-harbouring cloths are involved).

Kitchen surfaces and general cleaning If I need to clean the kitchen surfaces I half fill the sink with hot water and half a cup of bicarb, grab an e-cloth and get to work. Sometimes I just drop a couple of drops of neat tea tree oil on to the surface or on to an Enjo mitt and clean up that way. If the surface is greasy, Julie from Living Clean advises: 'Treat oil with oil. Mix a little olive oil with some lemon juice and use a rag to apply it to the surface – the oil will get the grease moving and the natural acid in the lemon will cut through the dirt.'

For hardy general cleaning, I like Pierre d'Argent (from **www.lemonburst.co.uk**), a natural eco-friendly 'paste' of 100 per cent natural biodegradable elements including soap flakes, vegetable fat, glycerine and scented oil. Excellent for use on cookers, stainless steel, brass, leather, tiles and grouting and generally awkward stuff.

Drains It's undoubtedly not a pleasant job but we're encouraged to regularly clean drains. Rather than caustic soda, opt for a natural way of maintaining and unblocking drains. Flush them out regularly using half a cup of soda crystals, half a cup of white distilled vinegar and a kettle full of hot water.

Earth Enzymes make a vegan drain opener that's safe for septic tanks. Buy it from **www.spiritofnature.co.uk**.

For sinks, pour plenty of boiling water down the plughole, and then add two cups of bicarbonate of soda and an equal amount of white distilled vinegar into the plughole until it begins to fizz. Get a good old-fashioned plunger on the case too.

Bathrooms If the bath is very grubby I use a Neem Household and Bathroom Cleaner containing neem and citrus from **www.junglesale.com** (neem is fantastically antibacterial). For the ceramic sink I find nothing makes it sparkle like a squeeze of old lemon.

Taps To remove limescale on taps, soak a cotton wool or fabric pad in white distilled vinegar and wrap it around the taps. Cover it with a plastic bag and then hold in place with an elastic band. Leave the vinegar to work for a couple of hours and then wash it off.

Ovens, hobs and pans To clean the cooker, an absorbent microfibre cloth or mitt and perhaps a bit of bicarb really is all you'll need. I'm talking about the hob really – no one cleans inside their cooker that often, do they? I'd avoid regular commercial oven cleaners – the last time I tried one, about 15 years ago, I couldn't cook a meal for weeks because the chemical whiff penetrated everything.

The Vitreous Enamel Association recommends Astonish (**www.astonish.co.uk**), who according to the blurb make incredibly versatile cleaning pastes that are suitable for the really dirty jobs and will cut through grime, grease and tough stains inside the oven and on the hob. It contains no animal products, is non-acidic and non-caustic, has no fumes and is biodegradable.

It's always a good idea to loosen off the grime in the oven by leaving a big pan of hot water and bicarb in there on a low heat. It will soak up some of the smells and the steam should loosen some of the grease.

Bicarbonate of soda can be spread liberally inside a fairly grimy oven, dampened with water (use a spray bottle) and left overnight. In the morning you'll need a couple of cloths to remove the gunk and wipe down the white residue, but it beats your roast dinner smelling of scary chemicals fumes any day. Bicarb and water works for just about all pans too.

Similarly if you've decided to purge your home of fizzy drinks you can simmer a pan of cola on the hob to loosen the gunk, very odd whiff, that one! I've also heard that boiling cinnamon is good, more for the Christmassy aroma.

Marble and granite Howard Naturals (from www.shinypad.co.uk) make a granite and marble cleaner, non-acidic, non-abrasive and without, they say, 'unwanted chemicals'.

Wooden furniture Avoid regular furniture polish, as it contains highly toxic chemicals. Look at www.auro.co.uk for natural alternatives or use natural beeswax for wood.

You can make your own furniture polish by mixing olive oil with white distilled vinegar – 3 parts vinegar to 1 part oil.

Glass mirrors Back to the old style again: newspaper and vinegar really do work a treat.

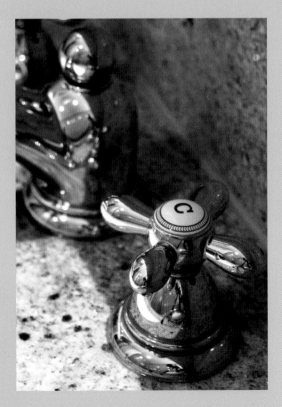

An eco-commercial option is the certified organic Window Spa from Natural House (www.natural-house.co.uk).

Plastic Bicarbonate of soda mixed with a little water will clean most plastics. It's especially good for baby bottles and bowls (though I'd highly recommend switching to glass because of the problem with plastics leaching hormone-disrupting chemicals).

Silver I can't pretend I own much, if any, silverware but I have it on good authority that tomato sauce will shine it up a treat. The professionals apparently use a metal sheet to clean silverware and a domestic version is called Silverstar. You place the sheet in your sink, and cover it with salt, boiling water and the silverware that needs cleaning. It can be used over and over and requires no chemicals – brilliant for around £15 from www.guardianecostore.co.uk. A paste made from bicarbonate of soda and dishwasher liquid (eco-friendly, of course) will polish up chrome.

Electrical stuff For cleaning clocks, cameras, computers, TVs and all electrical items your best bet is a dry microfibre cloth or soft small brush. Usually it's just a case of regularly getting rid of the build-up of dust. Ionisers (see page 139) will help too.

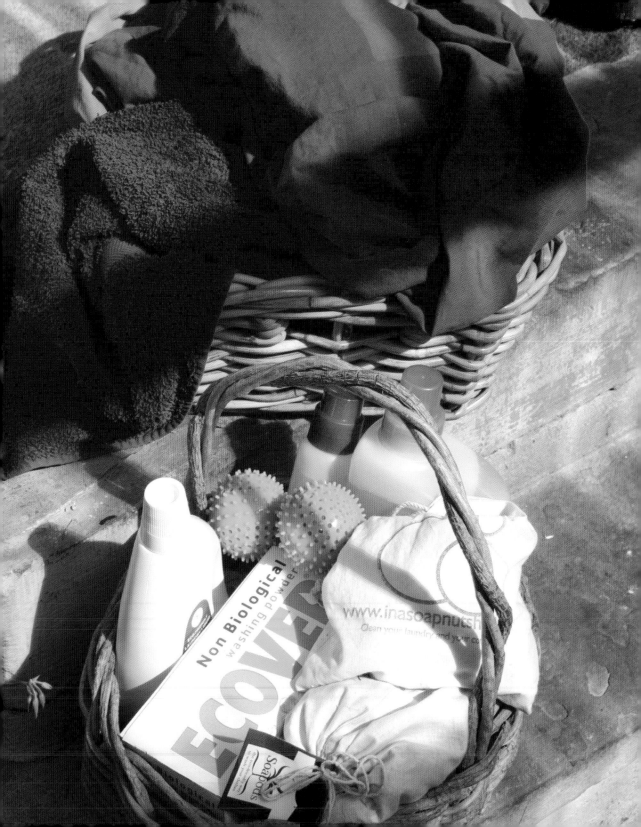

2 Laundry

This is one area where you will definitely feel called upon to make some changes and reduce that carbon footprint. Although it's widely accepted now that it's okay to wash at 30 or at most 40 degrees, and regular washing powders are singing loud and proud about their eco credentials because they want it known that their detergents are effective at lower temperatures, sadly while that might help save energy, it certainly won't help save your skin, or the fishes for that matter.

The Centre for Integrated Environment and Toxicology in Denmark found that in the UK alone, we do 17 million washes per day, each one draining 50 litres of water into the earth.

If 98 per cent of people are using commercial laundry detergents, that's a staggering one million and sixty thousand tons of detergent. The same study found that we use one million tons of fabric softener too. So that equates to a tragic waste of pure water and an accumulation of yet more chemicals into the environment that are slow to biodegrade.

Of course, one option is to do less laundry but that's unrealistic for many people (although I do think many items of clothing can be worn more than once before needing to be washed, underwear and children's clothes aside), but if you want to continue using powder or liquid detergents, use eco-friendly products. Most of the companies already referred to make a laundry detergent. Ecover do an excellent Integrated powder, and the Perle de Provence laundry liquid is good too.

But how much more creative, kind to our skin, infinitely cheaper and generally more fun are laundry balls and soapnuts? Oh, how passionate I've become about them! They are totally eco-friendly and as there's no extra rinse required, we use less water too.

LAUNDRY BALLS

Laundry balls are supercharged with ionised pellets that change the molecular structure of water, and draw dirt and grime away from clothes. Pop two of them in the drum of the washing machine with the laundry and that's it. They save water because there's no need for a rinse cycle, because they don't create 'soap' that needs to be rinsed off. There's also no need for a fabric softener – they do that all in one. For a fragrance you can add a couple of drops of essential oil to the detergent compartment or get a laundry spray from **www.homescents.co.uk**.

I've tried most of the laundry ball brands. The hard plastic casings tend to break and then they 'shed' their pellets and inevitably you find yourself chasing them across the kitchen floor and need to refill. The best I've found are Aquaballs (**www.aquaball.com**). Their casing lasts a lot longer. The pack costs around £15 and includes a stain remover and extra pellets.You can also spend a little more, to the tune of £35, for Ecoballs (**www.ecoball.com**). They claim to do at least 1,000 washes, so at approximately 35 pence per wash that's a good saving on regular detergents.

Of course, to conserve energy we must only do our washing when we have a full load. However, one tip is not to overfill your washing machine, as it's thought part of the benefit comes from the 'pounding' process, so the balls need some space to 'agitate'.

SOAPNUTS

These are little wonders of nature and I want you to remember if I'm the first person to introduce you to them – I want the glory! Soapnuts are an entirely renewable resource, technically berries rather than nuts, from the Sapindus mukorossi plant, which bears fruit for about 90 years. They have been used for thousands of years in India and Nepal. Initially you had to buy the whole nut and crack it, but now it's very easy to buy a bag of just the soapnut shells – the bit that you need.

You just put six to eight shells into a little linen drawstring bag and pop them in the drum of the machine – that's it! Reusable for between three and six washes, and then straight on to the compost heap. One tip from me: I find that because I have a washing machine with a front filter (essential if you have small boys and their daddy who put clothing into the wash with all manner of stuff still in the pockets), the drawstring on the little linen bags that come with the shells seems to open itself up during the washing process and I'm left with less than clean washing and a front filter full of not just the usual pennies and tiny plastic soldiers but also my eight soapnut shells. For this reason I've taken to popping them in a thin sock tied at the top – no escaping!

I really do find soapnuts keep my coloured washing brighter than laundry balls or detergent. Whites are pretty white too, though if you are a 'sparkling bright white' fan, you'll need to treat stains first and cheat with a bit of eco laundry bleach.

Soapnuts also make a great cleaning solution for washing the car and cleaning the house, and they're even great for washing your hair, but using them takes slightly more effort. For cleaning, boil a handful of soapnut shells in water, and then simmer for 20 minutes. The mixture won't look great – rather like 'brown water' – but for washing your hair you can whisk it up with a hand blender and create a really nice lathering 'soap' that's leaves it soft and silky.

You can get soapnuts for around £6 for 500g (which works out at approximately 15p a wash) from **www.ethicstrading.co.uk** or – worth it for the name alone – **www.inasoapnutshell.com**.

In some health shops now you can buy soapnuts as Soapods (**www.soapods.com**) and the company also make an excellent soapnut liquid.

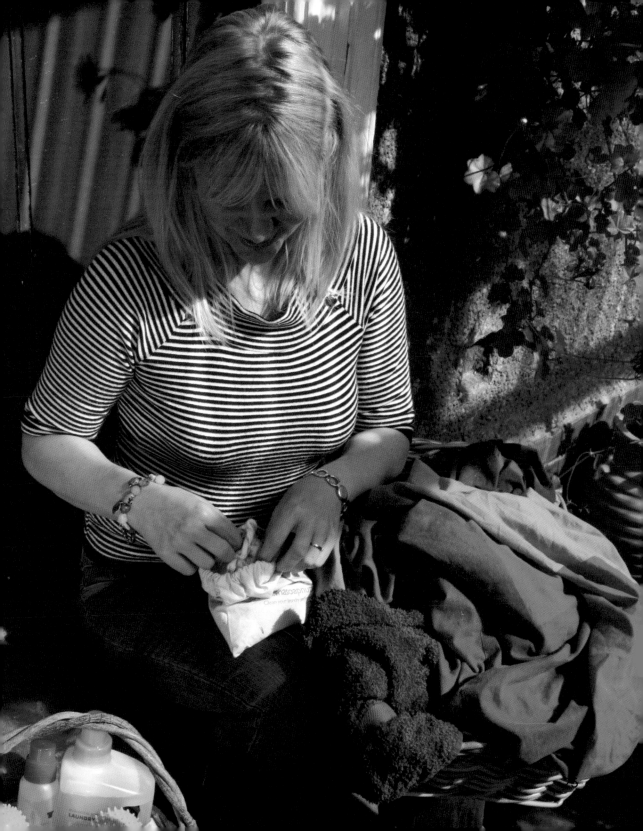

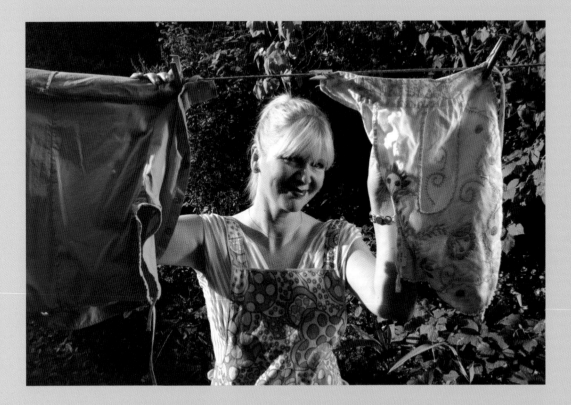

OTHER NATURAL ALTERNATIVES

There's a natural alternative to actual laundry balls and nuts and that's hypo-allergenic T-Wave laundry discs, available from www.goholistic.co.uk. They contain two types of 'activated ceramics'. They're meant to be very effective and a pack, priced at around £28, also includes a heavy-duty Natural Cleaning booster – a 947ml bottle of super-concentrated stain remover.

If you want to be super old-style, just mix a cup of finely grated soap with just under a cup of washing soda that contains no phosphates and biodegrades easily. Buy it in Boots or in

bulk from www.dri-pak.co.uk. Make the soap a natural one, though – Oliva soap from Holland and Barrett is good. To fragrance it, use a couple of drops of lavender or neat tea tree oil. Add a little borax to help with whitening.

You can also buy organic unperfumed soap flakes from www.natural-house.co.uk.

STAINS

If you must reach for the bottle, make it the excellent stain remover from Ecover, which I have found to work on clothing and on carpets.

Best of all for clothing stains, start with cold

water, as hot water will just set the stain in place. Food stains are usually sorted with just water and a bit of borax if needed. White distilled vinegar with bicarbonate of soda will sort out those awful sweat stains that appear on shirts (whether your deodorant is a natural one or not). Try making a paste with a dash of vinegar and bicarb in a little water, and hanging the shirts outside in the sunshine will definitely help.

For grass and oil stains, dab on eucalyptus oil.

Forget pouring white wine over a red wine stain: that's simply a waste of good wine. Try regular salt or soda water and always work gently inwards from the outside edge of the stain. Bicarb will absorb red wine from a carpet if you mix with a little water to make a grease-busting paste.

For all the above, treat the stain as soon as possible and always before washing. And for lots more tips see the excellent book *Natural Stain Removal Secrets* by Deborah L. Martin.

DRYING

When it comes to drying your washing, it has to be outside, doesn't it? I know our weather precludes that for a large part of the year but nothing beats the sight of a line of washing blowing in the breeze.

If you've got whites to dry, by the way, stick them out in sunshine with a quick squeeze of lemon juice directly on any unmovable stains, even ones you thought would outlive you.

In the winter months – and you can do this

if hanging washing outside isn't an option for you – I just use those old-fashioned clothes 'horse' type things. If you've got high enough ceilings, those old-fashioned overhead drying racks or pulleys are great; you can get them made from solid unvarnished certified pine with a manual pulley system. Years ago everyone had them, didn't they? Now in most trendy country cottages you're more likely to see copper pots and pans that are never used and a bunch of fake lavender hanging from them rather than the laundry they're designed for.

But what about when extra help is needed on the end of a plug?

Somewhere down the line since the mangle and the twin tub our mothers were sold the line about the 'tumble dryer'. Oh, and it's reverse action, allegedly so gentle to our fabrics. Everyone bought one, our electricity bills rocketed and we waited and we waited and still our clothes were not dry enough to actually wear.

Enter into my world the old-fashioned 'lid-top' spin dryer. It's similar to the contraption that squeezes the excess water out of your swimming costume before you stick it into a plastic bag at the gym. I first came across one when I needed to change bed linen for a whole household one Christmas. I saw one in a local junk shop for about £10 and thought I had nothing to lose. When I put my bed linen straight out of a 1400 spin into it I must say I didn't expect much to happen; the pipe running hopefully into the sink seemed to yield nothing as I pressed down the top and leant against it while it vibrated 'desperate housewives' style. Then all of a sudden a

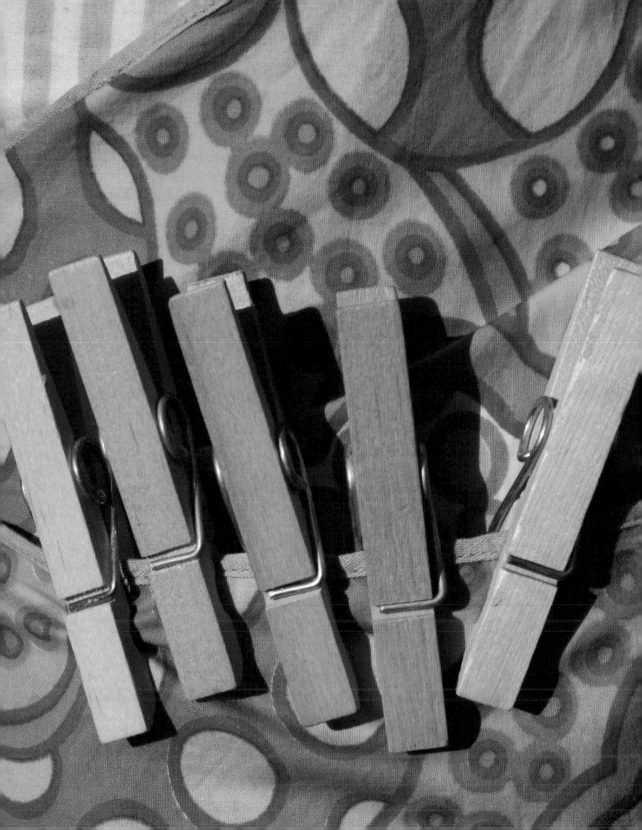

trickle of water came down the hose, followed by a veritable torrent! How could that be after a 1400 tumble dryer spin and an hour of costly electricity? My linen came out of the dryer bone dry – well, practically: I just needed to air the stuff as I would normally – and it had taken precisely two minutes

By the way, people often complain that their towels feel a bit 'rough' if they're not tumble dried. That's often down to what you're using to wash them in. Biological powders and detergents won't help and will certainly require a fabric softener. If you use laundry balls or soapnuts, you don't need to use fabric softener. If you live in an area with very hard water, as I do, though, you may still feel you need something else to help compete with the 'rough if not tumbled' feel of towels. One option is to add a spoonful of white distilled vinegar to the fabric softener compartment. I usually add a couple of drops of essential oil too. If you want to throw money at softeners – though not the ridiculous amount you waste in tumbling energy – then try the fabric softener from Ecover or one of the scented ones from Home Scents (**www.homescents.co.uk**), which offer eco luxury.

chemical whiffs. I was delighted, then, to find out about earth-friendly dry cleaning. Green Earth (**www.greenearth.co.uk**) uses a silicon-based fluid instead, which is thought to be non-polluting, and safe. Most Johnsons Dry Cleaners now offer this method, so although I'd say use dry cleaning as little as possible, when needs must opt for this more eco approach.

Think before you opt for dry cleaning, though. My friend Rosi, who is a stylist and TV costume designer, reckons a good percentage of clothes that say 'dry clean only' on the label can actually be washed at a low-ish temperature without any problem, and in fact doing so will considerably prolong the life of the garment. This is certainly the case with silk. By handwashing gently (being careful not to use harsh detergents) and rinsing in cold water there will be no damage whereas chemicals will break down the fibres in the fabric. You can also try steaming your clothes (see page 105 for more on electric steamers). Often a quick blast will freshen up a garment.

In any case, if you have your clothes dry cleaned, let them air for a while before putting them away in a wardrobe.

DRY CLEANING

Perchloroethylene (perc) is the fluid most often used in dry cleaning, and apart from the smell we can only imagine what it does to the rivers and seas once it has been 'discarded'. Somehow I just don't fancy that on my clothes, especially now my nose is attuned to unwanted

3 Food and drink

'Eat, drink, and be merry, for tomorrow we may diet.'

Harry Kurnitz, playwright

Back in the olden days, as I've commented on many times throughout this book, life was simpler, many households grew their own fresh produce and it was totally organic, not to be trendy – people then wouldn't have known what the word really meant – but because there were less potentially toxic pesticides available. The downside of this was that some of the precious vegetables fell by the wayside to the aphids or slugs, but what was grown was not only organic but fresh, with no food miles or pollution and of course grown in season. Our bodies were designed to eat foods that grew in our vicinity, in season, and I believe we've upset the balance of natural seasonal variety in our diets. The obsession we now have with eating strawberries in winter and mangoes flown in from Kenya all year round has contributed to a huge rise in packaging, fuel costs and potential contamination and reduction in nutritional value of the foodstuffs from roadside pollution and cold storage. Often produce labelled 'organic' doesn't always escape the same fate.

The difficulty is that even if you do source home-grown foods they're not always what they seem. Some supermarkets buy, for example, green beans grown by local UK farmers, and fly them out to other European countries to be trimmed, washed, packaged and then flown back to be sold as British-grown produce. Technically they are, but it's hardly helping the 'food miles' cause or enhancing their nutritional value.

Commercial foods labelled 'organic' may not necessarily be the most fairly traded, ethical or even healthiest item we could be eating. The label may simply mean it contains only 10 of the normally allowed 25 pesticides. Different accreditation schemes mean that produce can still have encountered a considerable amount of pesticides, chemicals and generally un-eco treatment but still make the grade to be labelled organic.

Without doubt the Soil Association (**www.soilassociation.org**) demands the most conclusive and stringent form of testing and accreditation for organic foods, and it offers advice and help to farmers and growers too. It has some rivals in other areas, such as organic skincare and beauty products, but still remains one of the most regarded accreditors.

Without wishing to scare you half to death I suggest you read *Not on the Label: What Really Goes into the Food on your Plate* by Felicity Lawrence to help you make your food choices. It's a great idea to be armed with the knowledge of fair trade and ethics when it comes to food manufacture and production

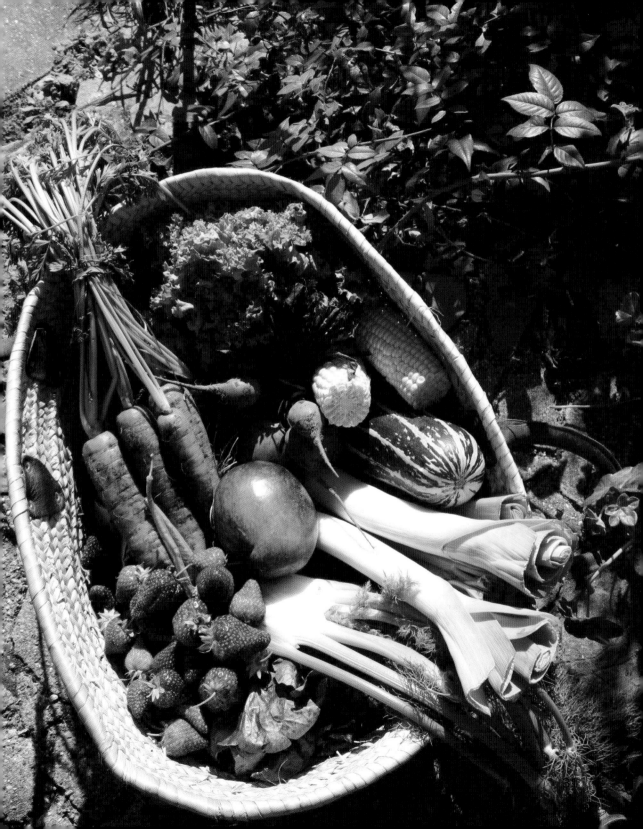

in the UK. Good old Hugh Fearnley-Whittingstall, too, has made a huge contribution to explaining everything about the food chain.

FRUIT AND VEG

I now seek fruit and veg that is locally sourced and grown without pesticides or chemicals. First stop: your own garden (see below) and page 145. The next best bet is local farm shops, farmers' markets and some health stores. Nowadays I'm not such a stickler for having to see that 'organic' label. Chat to sellers on farmers' market stalls and often you'll find that they do grow organically, but they aren't allowed to label their produce 'organic' unless they're able to fund and sustain full organic accreditation, which many can't. Thank goodness things are changing, though, and there is now a growing demand for locally sourced foods.

Of course, the growing trend for fabulous 'whole food markets' is taking off too, with shops like Whole Foods in Kensington, London, and across some of the bigger cities branches of Fresh and Wild and Planet Organic, but if you shop in these, check which of their organic produce is locally sourced. We need to put pressure on both the health shops and the supermarkets to buy from local farmers and growers. Nag your local supermarket too – they will listen to customer demands.

Farmers' markets are in abundance across the UK and there's been a massive rise in the popularity of organic vegetables. Remember that it takes typically 30 per cent less energy to produce organic food. It's the 'think global, act local' approach.

To find out about local farmers' markets and good local foods in your area, type your postcode into www.bigbarn.co.uk and www.farmersmarkets.net.

If you're lucky enough to live in the south-east, www.ethicalfoods.co.uk do the work for you. They source locally produced and organic foods that are fairly traded and deliver them to your door.

For vegetable box schemes across the UK, www.abelandcole.com and www.riverfordorganics.co.uk are excellent and you may also find a scheme more local to you. They vary in price and quality, so do some research. If you're thinking of ordering a weekly box scheme, ask a few neighbours if they want to get one too and agree a delivery day. Phone a company and ask what discount they'll give for three new customers in the same street!

Some supermarkets are now stocking organic veg boxes too. I tried the Tesco one and it's great value at £10 (at the time of going to print). Just make sure you know where the produce is grown and preferably when it was picked.

Consider too a shared co-operative scheme with others in your neighbourhood or with other parents at your children's school, etc. (see www.infinityfoods.co.uk). There are excellent models of community buying, especially for dried and non-perishable organic and natural goods, which save considerable amounts of money and travelling time.

For a reminder of what's in season,

see **www.eattheseasons.co.uk**.

If you want to get some wartime inspiration, see the wonderful book *Eating for Victory: Healthy Home Front Cooking on War Rations*, Foreword by Jill Norman (Michael O'Mara Books). It contains a nostalgic collection of original leaflets on healthy eating that were issued by the government and includes some great recipes such as Piquante Spinach and Savoury Potato Sandwich Spread.

EAT RAW

Of course, purists would say you have to eat a high percentage of your foods raw, as the cooking process destroys enzymes. For more information and some fantastic recipes, see *Raw Energy* by Lesley Kenton. See also *Living Foods for Radiant Health* by Elaine Bruce.

GROW YOUR OWN

With the interest in organic locally sourced produce, growing your own seasonal fruit and veg is becoming increasingly popular. There's been a huge growth in the number of people using allotments and in some areas there is a long waiting list to rent one from the local council.

If you want to grow your own but just can't face the whole 'waiting time', check out **www.rocketgardens.co.uk**. They'll send you an instant organic vegetable garden. It comes in the form of tiny established organic plants in biodegradable pots that can be popped straight into the ground, and within weeks rather than months you'll have fresh lettuces, radishes, strawberries – the lot. (See chapter 17 for more.) And even if you have only a tiny kitchen and no garden you can grow nutritious sprouts (see page 38) and some herbs on the windowsill.

You can also grow edible flowers and many more plants for food than the traditional vegetable range – see the website of Plants for a Future (**www.pfaf.org**). You'll be amazed!

If you have space to keep chickens, I'm told they're fantastically humorous pets and a source of wonderful organic eggs. Even inner-city dwellers can keep chickens. Go to **www.omlet.co.uk**, where you'll see the Eglu – an innovative 'chicken run'.

There's something very therapeutic about being even a little bit self-sufficient and even in my manic frenzy of always being busy I like the idea of 'slowing down'.

I enjoyed the book *In Praise of Slow: How a Worldwide Movement is Challenging the Cult of Speed* by Carl Honore (**www.inpraiseofslow.com**).

'The act of putting into your mouth what the earth has grown is perhaps your most direct interaction with the earth.'

Frances Moore Lappé, bestselling author and activist

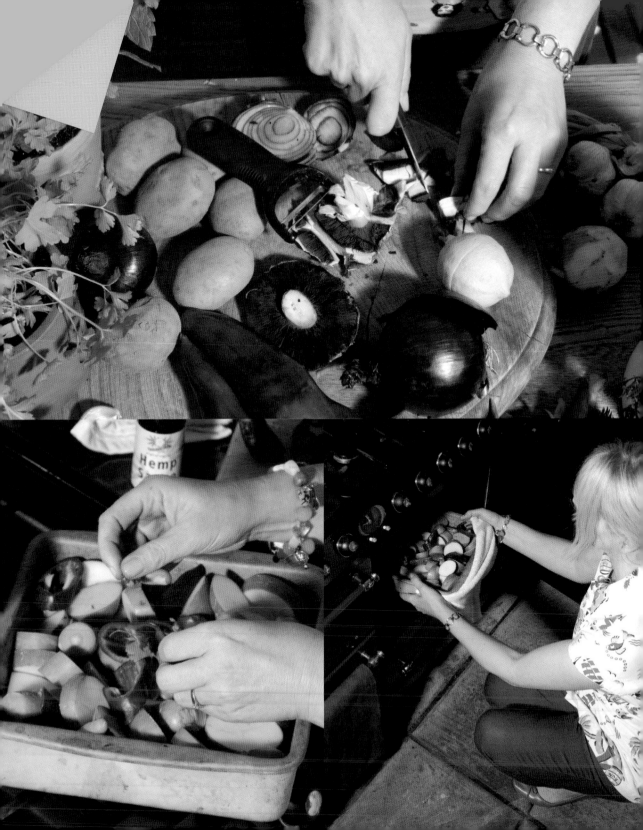

PREPARATION OF VEG

Much of the nutritional value of our fruit and veg is in their skins, but are the skins safe to eat?

Undoubtedly pesticides, herbicides and fungicides are not what's required in your healthy meal. If you buy a non-organic apple or cucumber, you'll note that it has a waxy appearance, not so the matt, slightly bruised finish of a home-grown one. That's because non-organic fruit and veg has often been coated with a mix that's made from petroleum-based products to improve the way they look and of course increase their shelf life. How scary that food can often outlive its packaging (I once bought a cardboard box of red peppers, forgot about them and when I discovered them, the box was starting to disintegrate but the peppers were fine).

The best advice is to wash all produce, but if you absolutely know it's organic i.e. you picked it from your own garden (well done you), a rinse and a scrub will suffice. If you don't know its source, wash with water with a dash of white distilled vinegar added, which will remove some but not all of the residues. You can also buy the organic Salad Spa fruit and vegetable wash from www.natural-house.co.uk.

Peel whatever must be peeled, of course, but remember that new potatoes taste just as good with their skins intact.

MEAT AND FISH

There isn't the space here to fully discuss nutritional issues or even to discuss the 'meat or no meat' argument. Sustainability of the planet, animal welfare and preservation of wildlife, plus personal health, are some of the reasons why it's prudent to eat less meat. For great animal-free foods go to www.bute island.com. They make the excellent 'sheese', which is 100 per cent dairy free but tastes fantastic on an oatcake.

Imperfection is OK by me of course. If you're going to eat meat or fish choose wisely. For meat, see if there is a local farm near you and ask if you can buy direct. If you're lucky enough to have an organic butcher near by, ask him to tell you all about his sources. Although I don't eat meat, my children do, and my local organic butcher, 'Gerard' of Boucherie Gerard in Mill Hill, North London, finds it highly amusing when I come in and ask him to prepare me a chicken or some organic minced beef without me 'having to look'. He's incredibly knowledgeable about where the meat is sourced and the conditions the animals are kept in. Some excellent organic companies who will deliver meat to your door include www.sheepdroveorganicfarm.co.uk and www.organicdeliverycompany.co.uk.

For meat and dairy, seek out sources from pasture fed animals, it makes a huge

'Zen does not confuse spirituality with thinking about God while one is peeling potatoes. Zen spirituality is just to peel the potatoes.'

Alan W. Watts, writer and philosopher

difference to the nutrient quality. See www.seedsofhealth.co.uk.

For fish, choose sustainable sources. Most of us are aware that blue fin tuna are endangered, but even cod and plaice are in short supply in some areas. Go to www.fishonline.org for info on which fish to avoid. Get into the habit of talking to your local fishmonger and make sure he can trace the source of his produce. It's always good, of course, if you can choose locally sourced options and look for the MSC certification of the Marine Conservation Society www.msc.org.

If you eat little fresh fish but want to take fish oils, you should still look for purity. I use Morepa Smart Fats, which contain EPA and DHA. Go to www.healthyandessential.co.uk.

Both organic fish and meat can be delivered to you by www.purelyorganic.co.uk.

WILD FOODS

Depending on where you live, check out local wild foods. 'Foraging' courses are becoming very popular, where participants walk to good local foraging sites and are encouraged to come back and devise a culinary delight with what they've found. www.wildman wildfood.co.uk is the wonderfully informative website of Fergus Drennan, who is a professional forager. Go on, take a look – admit it: you're curious!

After all, people were eating healthy nutritious foods from the wild long before we had the wheel, let along the supermarket aisle, so it makes sense that nature can provide all we need. Fairly recently experts have pieced together archaeological and historical evidence and concluded that a celebratory Stone Age meat and veg dish meal was likely to have consisted of fish gut soup and a roasted hedgehog, with a side order of dandelions, sorrel, chives and nettles...Yum! Dr Ruth Fairchild of Wales University led the research and found recipes that included a special nettle pudding. See also www.wildforest foods.co.uk, which supplies many London restaurants.

Roasted hedgehog is unlikely to be your thing or mine, but the message is: choose fresh, natural, in-season foods and avoid processed foods as much as possible, not withstanding being imperfect of course.

OILS

See page 86 in the section on Personal Care for my take on coconut oil, the finest oil for just about everything, but if you want a really vibrant herbal cooking oil how about this excellent recipe from Karon Grieves (www.dreamacres.co.uk), who grows organic herbs in her smallholding in Scotland and usually makes them into herb pillows:

Herbal Cooking Oil

Gather a good selection of fresh culinary herbs either from your garden or from local farmers' market/shops. A good choice is rosemary, savory (you will have to grow your own as this is not often found in shops – well worth adding to your garden, though, as it is great with veggies, especially beans), sage (not too much, as this is a strong herb), marjoram, basil, mint (just a little) and thyme.

Don't bother chopping the herbs, but do bash them a bit with a rolling pin to bruise them and release their precious oils. Now pack a large jam jar with a good mixture. You can add a few peeled cloves of garlic if you like. Fill the jar with olive oil. Screw on the lid and set aside in a cool dark place (a kitchen cupboard is fine) for 2–3 weeks.

Strain the oil through a sieve and pour into a pretty bottle, and keep it handy by the cooker. This oil is wonderful as a base for many dishes, from eggs to meat dishes and all sorts of fabulous veggie grills. It is also perfect for adding to salads and pasta dishes – a touch of flavour without too much effort.

SUPERFOODS

There's been a lot in the press about superfoods but there is no definitive list. Really, it's just a buzz word for foods that have a particular health-giving benefit. Most published lists of superfoods seem to include fresh foods that are high in nutrients, boost immunity, improve energy levels and that are proven to be anti-ageing.

Examples of foods often given the superfood accolade include oats, honey, certain types of meat and fish, all fresh veg and some herbs and spices, even tea, wine and chocolate feature in some superfood lists (with reservations), dried fruits including prunes, which are incredibly high in anti-oxidants, and just about all fresh fruits. Blueberries (the king of fruits) are top of my list.

Getting your daily quota of essential fatty acids (omega 3 and 6) is crucial. For this reason in addition to eating oily fish, it's a great idea to eat lots of nuts and seeds, which are also included in any good superfoods list. Get used to liberally sprinkling a mixture of seeds on to your cereals and salads. A great appetiser is a few blanched almonds lightly toasted without oil with just a dash of sea salt and fresh finely chopped chillies. You can also add hemp and flax oil, both a good source of essential fatty acids, to smoothies if you can't face taking them off the spoon.

I've waxed lyrical about sprouting seeds in previous books and I'm sure if you've vaguely heard about them but never tried them you'll at this point be saying, 'Oh please – give me steak or an omelette and stop being such a hippy.' I too used to find it hilarious that my flatmate would strain out her little muslin-covered jar twice a day and after four days tuck into her own home-grown crunchy sprout salads. But I'm older and wiser now, and having read about the nutritional benefits of sprouts and tried them myself I am now a convert. Don't get confused as my friend's student son did eat copious amounts of Brussels sprouts, which have an entirely different 'windy' outcome! Basically sprouts are seeds and pulses that are newly germinated, so they're packed full of nutrients, antioxidants, vitamins, minerals and enzymes, which of course would be destroyed in the cooking process. If you eat them regularly they can boost immunity, strengthen and revitalise you, and relieve stress and tiredness.

It seems as though it will be a huge alfalfing faff to grow sprouts, but really it's simple. Everyone can remember back to when they grew mustard and cress on a bit of blotting paper at school and the theory is the same. There are lots of starter kits available, and you can get everything to do with sprouting, including wheatgrass sprouters and juicers, as well as some great advice from Living Foods in St Ives in Cornwall **www.livingfood.co.uk**. If you get a chance to visit, make sure you taste all the wonderful combinations on offer and treat yourself to their sprouted salad with feta cheese for lunch. Add a few drops of hemp salad dressing too. Perfect.

If you're on the move and just want to buy a bag of ready-sprouted seeds to add to your sandwich, Holland and Barrett stores sell nice bags of Aconbury mixed sprouts and alfalfa sprouts.

When it comes to wrapping up sandwiches, by the way, ditch the plastic sandwich bags and use folded greaseproof paper or, even better, reusable containers with lids.

CHOCOLATE

My friend Michelle regularly reminds me that chocolate comes from a bean, which is in theory a vegetable, which means it's entirely reasonable to consider it one of your recommended five portions of fruit and veg every day!! I can't advocate that, but she's not that far off the mark so long as you opt for high-quality chocolate. Aim for a high cocoa solid ratio – at least 70 per cent if possible to get the most nutritional value – and make sure it's certified organic and Fairtrade.

The Day chocolate company campaign for Fairtrade and make Divine chocolate (**www.divinechocolate.com**), which is exactly that – divine. Organica is another excellent one and comes in some great flavours from **www.venturefoods.co.uk**.

I've recently become a fan of dairy-free chocolate; I'm not a vegan – it just tastes great. Nourish chocolate (**www.nourishme.info**) is a leading brand and has a 'female balancing' one, so called because it's fortified with omega 3s.

I'm also enjoying vegan raw chocolate (cacao), which contains no milk, emulsifiers, hydrogenated vegetable oils, sugar, flavourings or chemical additives.

www.rawchocolatecompany.com Another UK company is Raw Intent (**www.rawintent.com**): their chocolate is delicious, and they also make Raw Chocolate Pie, which is just the best dessert ever, containing organic raw chocolate, yacon powder, nuts and seeds, and sweetened with agave nectar.

If you're craving something sweet, a healthy chocolate substitute is to eat an organic pitted date straight from the freezer.

For lots more on sweet treats, see my book *Imperfectly Natural Baby and Toddler*.

BREAD

I know that as a rule I'm telling you to reduce the 'stuff' in your life, and particularly the stuff you plug in, but unless you're a domestic goddess and are happy to spend time kneading and pummelling I'd say have a bread maker and use it daily. When you really look into the ingredients of commercially produced bread, even some of the brands that are labelled organic, believe me you will want to make your own and control what goes in. Don't be fearful of complicated weighing and measuring: after the first few loaves, we just learnt to chuck in roughly what's needed – a cupful of this and teaspoon of that, etc. The great thing is that you can choose your flour, and you can add honey instead of sugar, and seeds to increase the omega-3 levels. You'll find home-made bread will keep for only a couple of days at most – if you haven't eaten it all up while it is warm! It makes you wonder what's in the shop-bought stuff that makes it last for seven or eight days.

WATER

With the enormous amounts of energy used to store, transport and make enough plastic bottles for 50 billion gallons of water worldwide every year, bottled water is about as un-green as you can get. That's before you get into the possible dangers of the bottles themselves. Chemicals used in the manufacturing process can leach into the water and increase substantially over time, and some of this stuff has a shelf life of two years. Authorities suggest contaminants are within safety levels, but other reports say that there is simply not yet enough evidence on the long-term effects of contaminants known to be present in the bottles. Increased consumption of bottled water has been cited as a possible cause of increases in levels of food poisoning. That's easy to understand, if like me you leave a half-drunk bottle lying in a hot car all day.

But let's face it: we're always going to need a bottle of water on the run, so I'll look for one of the non-plastic eco-alternatives such as Belu mineral water (**www.belu.org**), sourced near the Black Mountains in Carmarthenshire. Their biodegradable bottles look exactly like any small bottle of mineral water but are made from corn and, as I saw rather charmingly on the 'blurb' of one, need to be stored in a clean, dry rabbit-free place. They can be commercially composted back to nature in about 12 weeks – wait for it – one million years faster than regular bottles.

There are also some great new developments from companies like Ecolean (**www.ecolean.com**), who make sustainable packaging that is chalk-based. It's already in use in Germany and hopefully by the time you read this you may in fact have your water or juice/yoghurt/milk in this biodegradable packaging. For recycling regular drinks cartons see **www.ace-uk.co.uk**.

Best of all, of course, if you're going to drink bottled water, is buy it in glass bottles, which you can then recycle or re-use.

For the health-conscious, there's also the much-publicised Deeside water. Scientists attribute the longevity of the royal family in part to this mineral water, which flows near Balmoral. The secret is apparently the combination of minerals it gathers as it filters through granite and peatland before being bottled. **www.deesidewater.co.uk** If you can't give up flavoured water, avoid the sweetened kind and opt for Carpe Diem (available in supermarkets), which is botanical water with no artificial sweeteners but containing natural fruit sweeteners.

I've saved myself a fortune by investing in a reverse osmosis water filter under my sink, which filters out lead, copper, arsenic, cadmium, chlorine, giardia, pesticides, salt, trihalomethanes, sulfates, cysts, fluoride, nitrates, as well as some bacteria and viruses. Mine was from **www.drydenaqua.co.uk**; see also **www.freshwatersystems.co.uk**. If you can only use a jug filter, keep your filtered tap water chilled and it will taste great, I promise. Change the filter regularly, though. You can then re-use your glass bottles and fill up from your own tap.

ALCOHOL

In my imperfection I like a drink now and then, but in recent years I've become very particular about what wine I drink. I finally realised that the number of chemicals in the average bottle of wine is hair-raising and I switched to drinking only organic. Even then, it's not 100 per cent of course, but now where possible I opt for Soil Association accredited and Fairtrade wine. A great company, which will deliver and which really knows its grapes, is Vintage Roots (**www.vintageroots.co.uk**).They also have a wealth of information about vegetarian and vegan wines: it makes interesting reading. There's also the excellent company **www.festivalwines.co.uk**.

Of course, there's the food miles issue to consider and sadly here my imperfection pops up again. While on a camping holiday with my kids (boy, do I now know that camping is the new rock and roll) I passed a tiny vineyard – sadly I wasn't in France, I was in Essex – and I wish I could declare that the bottle of wine I bought there was good, but sadly it was not even passable. So for me UK-produced wine is not an option – yet. You, of course, might brew your own or know better. And it's changing fast, I'm told, so check **www.english-wine-producers.co.uk**.

'To take wine into our mouths is to savour a droplet of the river of human history.' Clifton Fadiman, critic

Certainly I have friends who lovingly produce sloe gin every year, but please don't send me down that slippery slope...

Organic beer comes under the same kind of controls as organic food, and is increasing in popularity, with more and more options appearing on UK supermarket shelves. Hops aren't easily grown in the UK, so much of the organic stock is imported, brewers claiming that organic malts and hops leave no chemical residues to interfere with the fermentation process and that the use of fewer pesticides can lead to a grain with overall better brewing characteristics. **www.1516beer.co.uk** and **www.realale.com** have a good selection.

Cider is becoming much more popular again and my beloved Cornwall has the finest Cornish cider. The Soil Association has stringent guidelines for organic cider production, covering the process, additives and of course the apples. Helford Creek (**www.helfordcreek.co.uk**) has excellent apple juice and cider.

COFFEE AND TEA

Well, the operative word is imperfect. Caffeine is not ideal – we know that – but if you're going to indulge, at least make it Fairtrade. There's no excuse now not to have fairly traded coffee: we all know about the huge mark-ups in coffee shops on unfairly traded coffee. Do your bit: buy Fairtrade, and organic. Look for a list of suppliers and cafés at **www.fairtrade.org.uk** or **www.cafedirect.co.uk**.

There's also great organic coffee that's fortified such as the excellent 'clarity' blend from Spava Coffee **www.fortifiedcoffee.com**.

Remember to put your coffee grouts on to the compost, and if you use paper filters chuck them on to the heap too.

There's a wealth of choice for organic Fairtrade teas. Clipper Teas (**www.clipper-teas.com**) and Steenbergs (**Steenbergs.co.uk**), for instance, do excellent Fairtrade and organic selections.

It's simple to infuse your own herbal teas too. To make refreshing mint tea, just pour hot water over a handful of fresh mint, leave for a couple for minutes, then strain and pour. Add a slice of lemon for a 'zing'.

SOFT DRINKS, SMOOTHIES AND JUICES

Mass-produced fizzy drinks and soft drinks are in my humbly imperfect opinion to be avoided at all costs. They have no nutritional value and usually contain copious amounts of artificial sweeteners and a cocktail of scary chemical additives. Fortunately the message is getting across. Several schools have banned fizzy drinks and seen an incredible improvement in the attention span of the children. If your children like fizzy drinks, wean them off them with pure apple juice or freshly squeezed orange juice mixed with sparkling water. You can also get 'healthy' carbonated canned drinks from Whole Earth in good supermarkets.

For organic apple juices, go to **www.helfordcreek.co.uk**.

You can of course make your own 'no

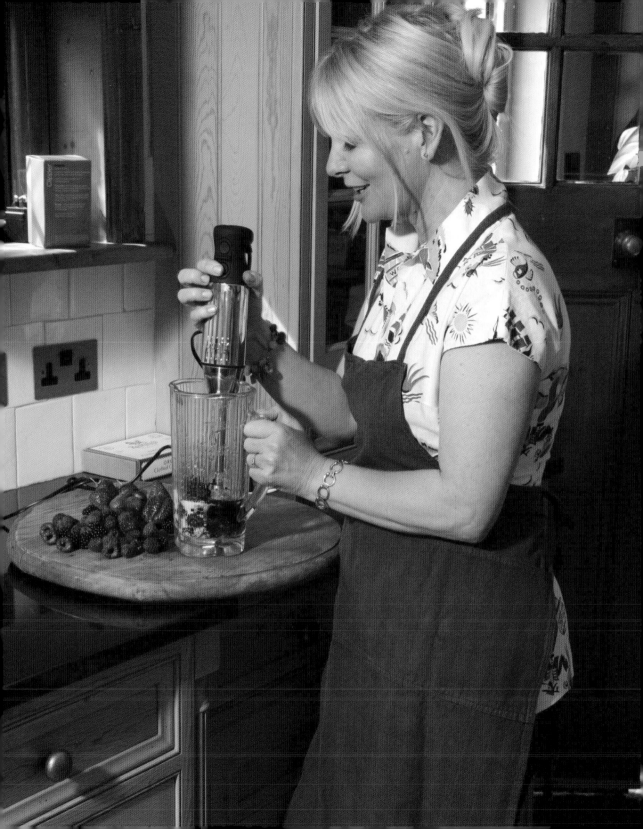

Smoothie

Here's a fantastic power-packed healthy smoothie with all the omega 3s you need. You can whizz it up in about two minutes flat with just a hand blender. Kids love its creamy texture and it's a great way of sneaking healthy oils into them.

Put slices of organic banana and blueberries, raspberries or any other soft fruit into a jug – avocado works well too. Add a dessertspoon of flax oil or hemp oil, a small handful of sesame seeds, pumpkin seeds and sunflower seeds, and three cups of oat milk, rice milk or natural yoghurt. You can also add manuka honey and even half a teaspoon of probiotic powder.

Plug in your hand blender and blend – it will only need about 30 seconds. Stand back as it whizzes or else you'll be sprayed.

Or why not make your own? If you already have a hand blender in your cupboard gathering dust, clean it up! To wash it, just rinse one end under the tap as soon as you've finished using it.

If you're harbouring a lovely juicer somewhere in your kitchen cupboards, get it out, clean it down and stick it in pride of place on your work surface. Without a doubt, juicing is the quickest and best way to get your five portions of fresh fruit and veg, plus all the power-packed enzymes you need. Keep a bowl of fresh organic fruits and veggies ready next to the juicer with a knife and chopping board and then it will remind you every day. If you are buying a juicer, look for one that cleans easily: it's important to clean up straight after you've drunk your juice, as nothing is worse than leaving it and then coming back to a festering juicer. Keep a small nailbrush just for cleaning out the awkward bits. The Champion Juicer has long been the champion but isn't cheap, although it has come down in price to just over £200. Moulinex also does great juicers, which are much more affordable, and the Phillips Wide Shute Juicer at around £79 takes even apples whole so saves on chopping time. For great advice on the best juicers and for some wonderful recipes, go to **www.juicemaster.com**.

waste' apple juice and your own old-fashioned lemonade or lemon barley water (for recipes, see my first book *Imperfectly Natural Woman*).

Prune juice is back in fashion too – it's fantastic for pregnant women and high in antioxidants. Get the freshly squeezed variety from **www.sunraysia.co.uk**.

For smoothies on the go, it's hard to beat Innocent smoothies (**www.innocent.co.uk**). My children also love the little pure fruit pouches from Ella's Kitchen (**www.ellaskitchen.co.uk**).

MEAL PLANNING

I must confess I'm an 'open the fridge and see what could make a meal' kind of gal, but those in the know tell me proper meal planning is the answer if you want to control a budget, make sure you always have the necessary ingredients, and of course avoid wasting food.

Go to **www.1click2cook.co.uk**, which helps you to devise a meal plan, and if you're on a tight budget, get the excellent book *Budget Meals: Eight Weeks of Delicious Dinner and Dessert Recipes* by Kimberley Saunders.

Don't forget the humble soup. Anything can be used up and made into a nutritious meal. The old nursery rhyme 'Pease pudding hot, pease pudding cold, pease pudding in the pot nine days old' expresses exactly that. Even the old porridge went into the soup and then got added to with various leftovers. I'm not advocating leaving your soup pan lying around for nine days but you get the drift. Soup is incredibly healthy and a great way to 'sneak in' foods that are really good for you but you may not wish to eat 'exposed', such as seaweed, nettles and the like.

COOKING AND KITCHEN EQUIPMENT

Once we've chosen our foods, how should we cook them? We should take into account energy use as well as taste. Remember, for instance, to use the right size pan and keep a lid on where possible, as the food will cook much more quickly.

> *'Only the pure in heart can make a good soup.'*
> Ludwig van Beethoven

Of course a steamer will retain the nutrients in your vegetables; and though I personally don't like microwaves and feel concerned about the changing of the molecular structure of the food, if you've got one it will certainly reduce the amount of energy used if you just want to reheat something (see also page 69).

When it comes to pots and pans, from a health perspective I'd say old style is best yet again. All my non-stick Teflon and aluminium pans have gone – I don't want to wait around to find out what the possible effects of their long-term usage are. Cast iron is excellent and although good quality makes like Le Creuset (**www.lecreuset.com**) aren't cheap, they're good value, as your grandchildren could still be using them long after you've gone. Check on eBay for bargains.

I've also recently become converted to the fantastic cooking stoneware range from **www.pamperedchef.com**. They're great for casseroles, pizzas, flapjacks and biscuits – anything really, and they require no oil and, incredibly, no detergent for washing up.

By the way, avoid putting aluminium foil in direct contact with food, as it's thought there can be a link between aluminium and Alzheimer's disease. Good old-fashioned baking sheets (greaseproof paper) will do the job, whether under the food or as a lid.

Amazingly kettles can use two-thirds as much energy each year as our cookers do,

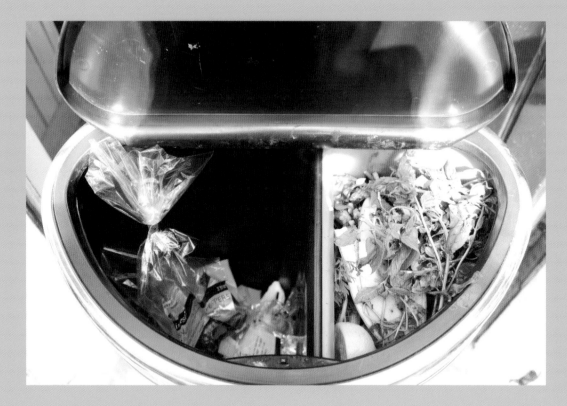

possibly because we almost always boil at least twice as much water as we need. Using a kettle on a gas hob uses half the carbon emissions that an electric one uses, but most of us are too impatient and imperfect to do this. Kettles with covered elements will reduce the use of power, as you can boil smaller amounts of water easily.

There are some eco kettles now that provide a marker or a gauge to enable you to measure the amount you need easily and these are said to reduce usage by approximately 30 per cent a year. You can also get a one-cup jug kettle, which boils the water in a staggering three seconds (www.ethicalsuperstore.co.uk).

KITCHEN WASTE AND COMPOSTING

Approximately 15 per cent of kitchen waste that's thrown away could actually be composted, and the catering industry is said to be throwing away a staggering 50 per cent daily.

If you live in a high-rise block, composting is unlikely to be a viable option for you, but nag your local council, if they aren't offering it yet, to offer a food waste collection. This means you can put all food waste in there and it will be taken for industrial composting, which will eventually be sold as green waste compost to local farmers. There may also be a Community

Composting project in your area that either gives or sells cheaply the compost back to households or uses it for local parks: see www.communitycompost.org.

If you have your own outdoor space, you'll want a compost bin. Check with your local council, because some will provide bins free or at greatly discounted rate. If you opt for a plastic one, make sure it's recycled plastic. For quick compost, try a 'rotating' composter such as the Blackwell compost tumbler around £55 (www.evengreener.com). Or make your own simple structure from bits of old wood. Just make sure it's got a lid or an opening for easy accessibility. It will just seem annoying if you can't get the lid off while carrying a heavy crock of waste or can't access it to give it a stir occasionally.

To that end, often people just have a heap. It will all rot down in time and there's a school of thought that says a compost pile open to the elements can regulate its wet-to-dry ratio rather cleverly. It will rot down more quickly, though, if you keep the heat in by laying on top of it a sheet of hessian-backed carpet or similar.

I was terrified of composting at first but eventually realised how easy it can be. Just sort out your waste – regular compost bins can take everything apart from cooked food, and do not add meat or fish, unless you have a wormery (more on that below) – and store it in a kitchen compost caddy. I use the Compost Crock from Lakeland (www.lakeland.co.uk), which holds a reasonable amount of waste and has a lid that contains a carbon filter to neutralise any odours. Every day or so I chuck it into the compost bin and, if I can persuade them, the kids stir it up from time to time. Basically the compost bin takes all uncooked leftovers, fruit and veg peelings, tea bags, egg shells, coffee grinds and of course dead flowers, plants and weeds. I've even been known to throw an old jumper in there. I like the look of Green Cones (from www.greencone.com), which take all food waste, cooked and raw, and even scraps of meat and fish, but they need to be sunk down into the ground so that they don't attract vermin.

If you have limited space, and especially if you have children, you might love a wormery. Yes, it's exactly that: live worms in a specially designed bin with a sealed lid. I've heard tales of them drowning, so be careful to get the levels of moisture right, but I know several people who love their wormeries, and indeed my little boy would be happy with one, as the whole process is much quicker than the regular composting. They take kitchen waste and, when the worms have done their thing, produce the most nutritious liquid fertiliser approximately six months after you get started. This can be diluted and used even for houseplants. See www.wigglywigglers.com.

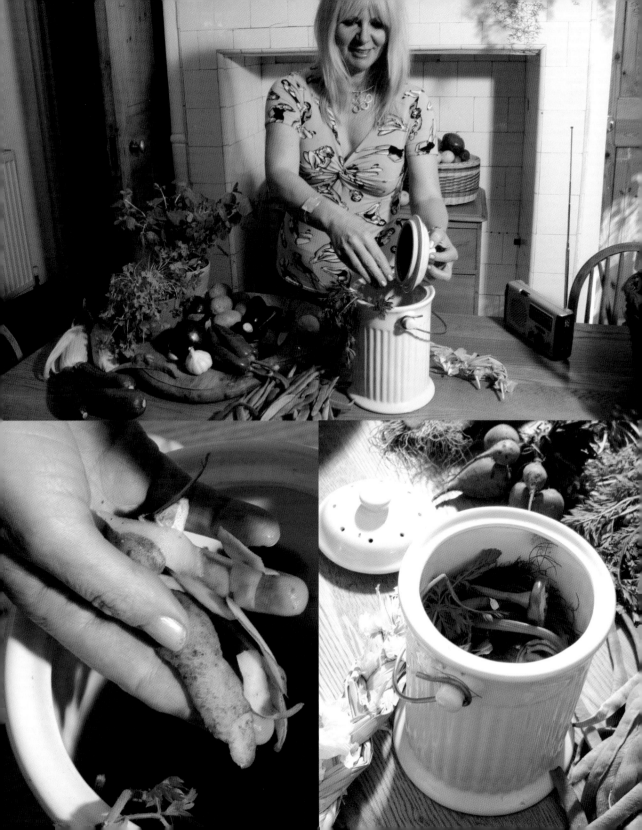

Imperfectly natural home Q&A

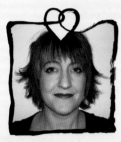

Alexandra Little
Full-time mum and have just set up 'Nappy Love', a website selling cloth nappies, organic clothing and natural baby toiletries.
www.nappylove.co.uk

Describe your home. Four bedrooms, detached with garden.

How many people live there? Five.

How would you describe your interior 'style' and furnishings? (E.g. cosy and comfortable, stylish and chic, antique, modern, minimalist etc.) Modern and neutral.

What does your home mean to you? It's a safe place to come home to where we are all comfortable just to be ourselves.

Have you attempted any eco DIY or modifications for a greener home? (E.g. solar panels, eco paints, wind turbines etc.) Was it worth it financially? No, we've been a bit put off by the cost.

How would your home rate for energy efficiency? What have you done to reduce energy usage? When you buy new appliances do you consider the energy efficiency? Reasonably efficient. We have good insulation; have changed to energy-saving light bulbs, turn things off as we go around. We recently bought the most efficient energy-rated fridge we could find and have a condenser dryer for 'emergencies' and we use the water from it to water the garden.

What ideas do you have for water saving? Turn the taps off when cleaning our teeth. Fit a water butt and share bathwater!

How 'eco' are your furniture, floorings and furnishings? Not at all, we had everything in place before we became more eco aware.

What cleaning/laundry/stain removing products do you use? For cleaning we use vinegar, bicarb, tea tree & lemon oil and Ecover Squirt. For washing, it's Ecover washing powder and white vinegar. Just about to try the much raved about soap-nuts!

If you could buy any one 'eco' gadget or item for your home inside or out what would it be? Some solar panels.

What kind of cookware do you use? Non-stick/cast iron? Stainless steel and ceramic.

What's your best tip for getting your fridge and larder stocked with good healthy food? Do you plan meals in advance, grow your own, shop locally?
I plan our meals about a week in advance and shop for what I need every few days.

Almost everything I buy is organic and local. Fruit, veg, dairy produce and eggs come from either a local farm shop or box delivery. I bulk-buy dried goods from Suma – much to my poor husband's horror: 'Where's all that pasta going?'
www.suma.co.uk

What about composting? Just ventured into composting, we have bought a bin from the local council so watch this space!

What do you regularly recycle? How? (E.g. door collection) Glass, cardboard, paper, tins and plastic. We have containers for each and my husband takes it to the recycling centre as our council don't do doorstep collections. Between that and cloth nappies, we have cut our rubbish down by two thirds.

If you have a garden, what are your eco tips? Soap suds from my Ecover or soapnuts to kill greenfly on my rose bush.

Do you have any 'alternative' pet tips? No pets.

Have you ever considered 'Feng Shui' for your home? Would love to but haven't done it as yet.

What are your views on the possible dangers of electro 'smog' wifi/emfs etc.? Have you taken any protective measures? Scares the life out of me since becoming more aware of the dangers! My first step was to buy some Green 8 Foils for our mobiles, cordless phone and baby monitor.
www.sheerprevention.co.uk

Do you know your carbon footprint and do you care about it? (Be honest!) Yes and I do care about it now I have a child of my own. We do what we can to minimise it but it scares me that some people think that by planting a few trees it makes it all okay – if only it were so simple!

How green are you – lime/olive? About the colour of avocado flesh and getting greener a bit at a time!

Do you have an imperfectly natural guilty secret? I tumble dry my little girl's nappies every so often so they're a bit fluffier for her bottom!

What would your dream home be like? A white cottage in the open countryside with a little white fence around it and a stream at the bottom of the garden!

What are your top three tips for a naturally healthy home? Ditch the chemical cleaning products. Use essential oils instead of commercial air fresheners and open your windows. Say thanks for your blessings every day – it makes your home a happier place.

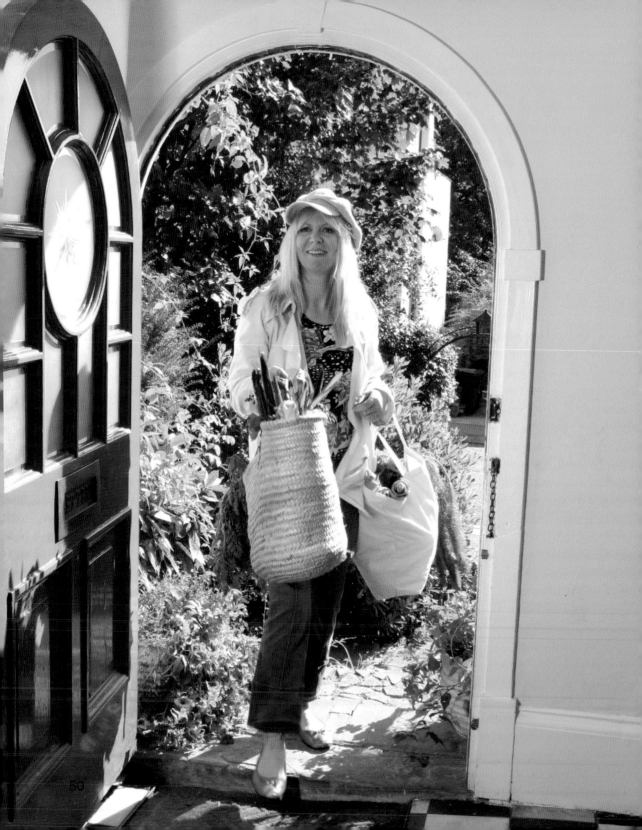

4 Recycling

> '*The waste of plenty is the resource of scarcity.*'
>
> Thomas Love Peacock, author

I remember that as a kid in the late 1960s, the 'pop man' would come around quite often, and in addition to selling us bottles of lemonade he would take back our empties. We had milk delivered daily and our empty bottles were always put out for collection. I don't think my mum would have dreamt of throwing a glass bottle into a bin; in fact, as kids we would knock on our neighbours' doors and ask if they'd like us to take their pop bottles back to the shop, as that way we kept the shilling. Even as a teenager I remember the rag and bone men. The name comes from the fact that along with old junk, they at one point used to collect cloth, and old bones for making glue.

Recycling is an old idea, so I don't know why we think we've suddenly invented it. Previous generations with their 'waste not, want not' lifestyles were pretty good at it and would have been appalled at today's 'guesstimate' that only 17 per cent of our recyclable waste is actually recycled. To many of them the word 'recycling' meant getting back on to your bike when you'd fallen off.

SHOPPING BAGS

In the olden days that bicycle would have had a nice wicker basket to carry the shopping. Baskets may be cumbersome but are infinitely preferable to the nightmare plastic shopping bags.

Since the 'bag for life' has become so popular there are now a wealth of branded and unbranded easily foldaway bags to carry your shopping in.

See www.bags2keep.co.uk, www.onyabags.co.uk and www.turtlebags.co.uk – so named because turtles coming to UK waters are increasingly mistaking discarded plastic bags for jellyfish and getting caught up in them.

Another stylish concept is the 'Trolley Dolly', a bag that contains 22 more strong but lightweight bags! From www.zpm.com.

The important thing is to remember to take your reusable bag with you. If we all keep

> '*Waste is worse than loss. The time is coming when every person who lays claim to ability will keep the question of waste before him constantly. The scope of thrift is limitless.*' Thomas A. Edison, inventor

51

buying more and more of them, meaning more need to be produced, we'll be undoing all the good work.

CONSUMER POWER RULES

Next time you want to buy corn on the cob, buy it on the cob, not under an expanded polystyrene and cellophane cover, but just in its own protective organic packaging, in the form of a skin. As nature intended, designed perfectly to protect the cob. A huge amount of fruit today seems to have suffered a similar fate and is sold shredded of its natural protection, cut into neat squares and placed in plastic containers. Selling fruit this way is great for increasing the profit of the retailers, as by adding value they can charge more for it and it also reduces their storage and transport costs, as well as prolonging shelf life. But it passes the buck of waste-disposal responsibility on to the consumer. If we take along our own reusable bags and buy from markets and farms, make choices in the supermarket and do not buy stuff in unnecessary packaging, sooner or later retailers will get the message. In their defence they will always argue that the customer gets what the customer wants, so make your demands known.

As I type this book, the letters on my computer keypad are wearing out at a rapid rate, to such an extent that I can't see some of the letters any more (I won't name and shame the manufacturer) and that's an 18-month-old computer. I'll soon have to add to the computer waste mountain again, by getting rid

of it and getting a new one, and that's unacceptable. I'll be making a complaint to the manufacturer, as well as asking for a free replacement. Now if a million people did that, manufacturers would have to think about making their products last slightly longer. We could halve the mountain of dumped computer equipment in one fell swoop – oh, the power of the consumer! So let's reduce the amount we need to recycle in the first place by not buying products that are wasteful and over-packaged.

Our obsession with gadgets can only mean yet more electronic waste. Look to manufacturers that not only have good eco ethics but also have a quality and longevity reputation for their products. A good source is *Which?* (www.which.co.uk), which has been assessing companies and giving independent information and recommendations for years.

You'll be aware of the The Waste Electrical and Electronic Equipment Directive (WEEE Directive) which aims to make the manufacturers and distributors of products responsible for free recycling.

My motto is keep the pressure up – be discerning with your buying power and let big business know that reducing waste really is a joint effort.

Signing up to the Mail Preference Service (www.mpsonline.org.uk) will help reduce junk mail. You can also register the name of the previous owner of your house to ensure that you don't receive their junk mail.

GET INTO THE HABIT

Our intentions are good, and I think that as a nation there really has been a huge shift in our awareness, but it's not an option to claim imperfection and then do nothing. It'll take us all a while to change the status quo, so in the meantime my best suggestion is make recycling fun and therapeutic. Children and schools are leading the way with this, and it's a great ongoing pursuit for them. My seven-year-old will absolutely not let me discard anything without thinking, and my darling husband also helps (while suspecting it all ends up in China).

On that issue by the way, there's no dispute that China drives the global waste trade, for more information see **www.wrap.org.uk**.

Without a doubt, we need more infrastructure in place in the UK for economically viable collection, sorting and recycling. Meanwhile do your bit, get yourself some 'sorting bins' and just get into the habit of chucking in different directions – after you've thought carefully whether the item could be composted, given away or re-used of course. (Wherever possible buy containers that are refillable. If you buy Ecover cleaning products, for example, they are designed to be refilled, so call 08451 302250 or go to **www.ecover.com** to see if there's a 'filling station' near you.)

When it comes to household paraphernalia, remember that 'one man's junk is another man's treasure'. So instead of dumping, let's find another good home for our unwanted items that can't be recycled and save them from landfill. See eBay (**www.ebay.co.uk**) if you want cash of course, but also think of Freecycle (**www.freecycle.org**.). This is a global organisation with lots of local groups. It's becoming so popular that you may even find there's a waiting list to join. Members post details of an item to give away and you post a message back saying 'yes please'. No postage or parcelling up involved: the item is free to the agreed person, who comes and collects it. You can also post a 'wanted' notice, but don't be greedy. I once saw a 'wanted' sign for a 'large family estate car with low mileage'!

A great nationwide site is **www.myskip.com**. It's a free version of eBay with lots of celebs adding their tips and ideas on recycling.

Have a good clear-out yourself and make some cash at a car boot sale. For books, go to the excellent **www.readitswapit.co.uk**, which does what it says on the tin, or if you want to make a small amount of cash for your books, sell them via **www.greenmetropolis.co.uk**.

You can also swap just about anything, from houses, cars and bikes down to DVDs and toys, at **www.swapxchange.org**.

Also, remember your creativity: some

'He had that curious love of green, which in individuals is always the sign of a subtle artistic temperament, and in nations is said to denote a laxity, if not a decadence of morals.' Oscar Wilde

wonderful art comes from junk. Perhaps it could be you winning the next Turner Prize for your installation – an innovative 'Womble-esque' use of everyday things. For inspiration, check out www.junk.com, where you can see some wonderful examples of artistic endeavours and new uses for old objects.

A great 'scrapbook warehouse' resource for kids is Children's Scrapstore (www.childrensscrapstore.co.uk). Local businesses donate all their unwanted fabrics, stationery items and all manner of colourful kit, and you or your children's school or playgroup can collect as much as you like for free (some branches have an annual membership fee).

Remember that even really old woollens can go on the compost, and old shoes and kids' clothes can be stuffed into clothes' banks, often situated in supermarket car parks. Charity shops aren't choosy, and donating makes you feel just as good as 'gaining a few quid'; they're useful when you want a clear-out and just can't be bothered to eBay or advertise. With linens and blankets, underwear and warm clothes, remember that your local church or homeless charity may be grateful for them.

Most of all think first before deciding to replace with 'new'. A friend of mine runs a small hotel and prides herself on being 'carbon neutral'. When she was seeking her 'hotel star rating' an inspector noted that her curtains were sun bleached and advised her to buy new ones. My friend disagreed and pointed out her ecological view, to which he was taken aback, saying he had never before heard such an argument! She got her star rating anyway.

A NEW MINDSET

It wasn't all that long ago that people darned their socks, mended their clothes and repaired their worn out toys and furniture. Sadly, most of us won't go back to that as this is a disposable society but even if we no longer 'make do and mend', before buying any new item, look first to see if someone has been innovative enough to create a recycled version. A whole industry has grown up now around recycled items. You can now buy bags made from plastic bottles and car tyres, tableware made from recycled Tetrapaks and any manner of paraphernalia that has been lovingly crafted from something else. A great source of inspiration for new ideas are the catalogues produced by the online eco stores such as www.greenerstyle co.uk and www.thegreenstoreonline.co.uk. These are often the frontline for eco innovations.

MORE IDEAS FOR RE-USING

Clothes

Fortunately I'm a big follower of charity shop chic. Always give your old clothes to charity shops (but for shoes and kids' clothes, see page above), and if you have something really unusual, see if a local fashion college would like it. For funky recycled clothes, check www.junkystyling.co.uk.

Tools and electrical equipment

Whenever you buy new tools, electrical equipment or the like, give away your old one to a friend or to an organisation who can make use of it. Tools for Self Reliance (**www.tfsr.org.uk**) have volunteers who will collect your old tools locally.

Computers

Tools for Schools (**www.tfs.org.uk**) supply computers for schools. Computer Aid (**www.computer-aid.org**) will send them to developing countries.

Furniture and household items

Some councils are happy to take unwanted furniture and household items to furnish community properties or resell. Also contact Furniture Re-use Network (**www.frn.org.uk**), who can link you up with local groups who restore furniture for people who need to furnish properties cheaply.

Paint

An amazing 20 per cent of the total amount of paint we buy every year is unused. Donate your half-opened tins to Community RePaint (**www.communityrepaint.org.uk**).

Tyres

Find a local garage or independent mobile mechanic who is willing to repair car tyres or give them a re-tread. Several companies now make new products such as shoes from tyres. **www.vegetarian-shoes.co.uk**

Mobile phones

Go to **www.foneback.com**. They will take your phone and recycle it. Also charity shops will take them off you (you don't need your SIM card).

Spectacles

Often your local optician will accept these, so check whether yours has a recycling facility. Otherwise some charities such as Vision Aid can make use of them.

In the workplace

Worktwice (**www.worktwice.com**) will arrange collection from offices of plastics, paper and electronics for recycling. Go to **www.recyclenow.co.uk** for some great tips and ideas. See also **www.wasteonline.co.uk** for more suggestions

There are some excellent books to help you much further with all of this. For a humorous but also inspirational approach, see *Diary of a Reluctant Green: Can you Save the Planet and Have a Life?* by Richard Hallows. See also *Make Do and Mend: Keeping Family and Home Afloat on War Rations*, foreword by Jill Norman.

'Nothing is cheap which is superfluous, for what one does not need, is dear at a penny.'

Mestrius Plutarchus, biographer

5 Heating, lighting and energy-saving

HEATING

Energy-saving is the kind of thing I wish I'd been taught and tested on at school, along with how to floss my teeth. There is much we can do to save on bills and energy consumption, and new technology is progressing in leaps and bounds.

Lowering usage is the most meaningful thing we can do most quickly and with the most impact.

It wasn't that many years ago when the average home was not centrally heated. I remember the three-bedroom council house my grandparents lived in being freezing in the winter months – so much so that I was actually afraid to run upstairs to the toilet and would wait as long as I could by the open fire. What bit of heat the fire generated would go flying out of the draughty old windows, which weren't double glazed, and when hot water was needed my gran used to have to boil the copper – a huge great contraption in the middle of the kitchen floor – and then carry buckets of water through the lounge and up the stairs to fill the bath. In my own home a few streets away my parents had the luxury of an immersion heater and an electric fire but still no radiators.

I know – I can hear you saying, 'That's nothing – we lived in a cardboard box, etc.' I'm not trying to do that 'life was better then' thing, but these days we are so mollycoddled in our warm centrally heated triple-glazed homes with our whirlpool baths, power showers and even patio heaters for the autumn that we sometimes forget that it is also possible to pop on a jumper if you feel chilly. Yet again by just spending a little amount, going a bit old style, and changing a few habits, you can make huge savings. If you're not at the stage of installing solar panels or a new boiler, or designing your own eco-build – and let's face it, most of us aren't – there's still an awful lot you can do to be energy-efficient.

You may want to do a home energy audit calculation. Resurgence offer an online one at **www.resurgence.org**.

Thermostats

Make sure your radiators have individual thermostats so that you can turn them off in rooms that are not in use, and think old style

'The earth is like a spaceship that didn't come with an operating manual.' Buckminster Fuller, architect, inventor

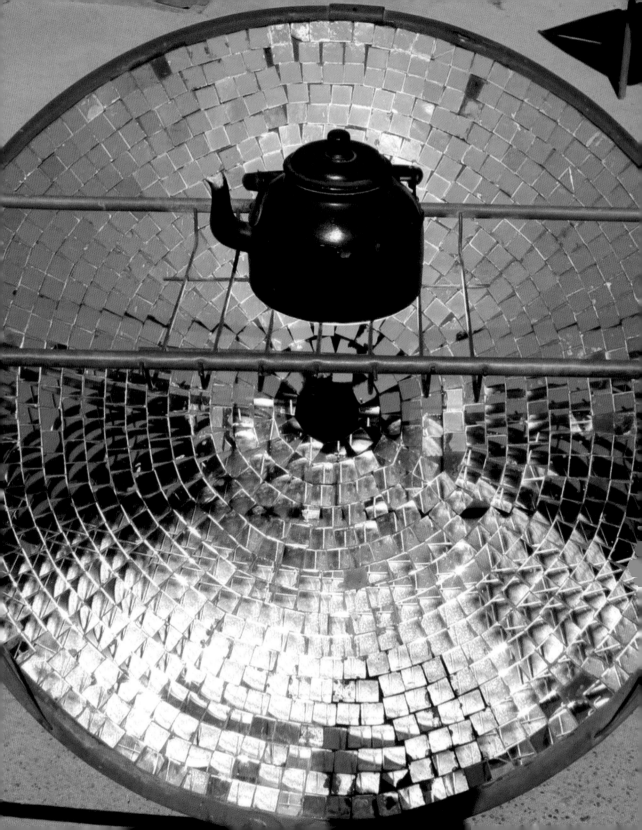

again with the insulation behind the radiators. Years ago we used to put tin foil behind them and it wasn't actually such a way-out idea. You can now buy ready-made radiator panels that are like padded foil.

I've turned my boiler temperature down one notch. A one-degree change can save you 10 per cent on bills. And while you're there, it's worth getting the boiler checked out. A simple service will not only reassure you on safety but could increase efficiency. If you're switching from a conventional boiler it's worth investing in an efficient condensing boiler. It's thought an average semi detached home could save £150 annually.

electricity. (An acre of poplar coppice after three years will provide approximately ten tonnes of wood each year to burn.)

If you're thinking of installing a new open fire, but don't have a chimney, one product I very much like the look of is the Flueless Fire system from CVO (**www.cvo.co.uk**), which is an open gas fire that not only looks lovely but burns so amazingly clean that you don't need a chimney or a flue. Up-market, stylish and efficient, and a far cry from the old 'gas log' fires.

'Chop your own wood, and it will warm you twice.' Henry Ford

Real fires

'You are a king by your own fireside, as much as any monarch in his throne.'

Miguel de Cervantes, novelist and poet

I am imperfect and I must confess I love sitting by a real open fire, so I need to assuage my guilt a little by at least using recycled logs from EBC Woodfuels (**www.ebc-ecofuel.co.uk**). If you use lots of logs, you can invest in a paper pulp log-making machine from **www.naturalcollection.com**. I know it sounds daft but you can make fire logs from newspapers, household and garden waste.

The best way to be self-sufficient (or as much as possible) is to have a renewable wood fire stove with back boiler for hot water and heating, and localised solar/wind (see page 64) for

Insulation

An amazing amount of heat is lost under doors, and through sash windows in need of repair, cat flaps and the like. If you have an older house, though, be careful not to seal everything up. That's not how old places work: they breathe and stay healthy through a balance of ventilation and heating, and if you disregard this you can unwittingly introduce condensation and damp problems. Good thick curtains work a treat – an amazing amount of heat vanishes through windows. You can spend a small fortune on good-quality curtains, so second-hand and reconditioned is a good option. The Curtain Exchange (**www.thecurtain exchange.co.uk**) have a good range. Wooden shutters are an excellent alternative too (**www.theshuttershop.co.uk**).

Don't forget your trusty old draught excluders too: make your own with a very long stuffed sock or buy one of the psychedelic snake draught excluders made with vintage fabric and filled with a natural biodegradable filling of buckwheat husks from Ecoutlet (**www.ecoutlet.co.uk**).

Loft insulation is fantastically eco-friendly in principle, in that the cheapest, greenest energy is the energy you don't use. Kit your loft out with eco insulation such as a paper-based one in bags from Natural Collection (**www.natural collection.com**). It's treated with a non-toxic fungicide, and is fire-tested to British Standard specs. Also there's cotton fibre insulation (recycled blue jeans) from Recovery Insulation (**www.recovery-insulation.co.uk**), which contains no melamine, phenolic resins or formaldehyde. The essential fungi and fire resistance is achieved usually by adding small amounts of low-toxicity boric acid.

It gives better sound insulation too, and best of all it's safe and doesn't give you that horrible (and potentially carcinogenic) itch when you're putting it down. A great eco option. Grants are obtainable, but don't rely on one, as it's a bit of a lottery actually getting them; you may find that councils want to have a say in your choice of insulation materials as well.

Of course, heat is lost through walls too – an estimated 35 per cent. Insulating walls is a pro job (be careful to check what materials they're using), but your costs should be recovered within five years. An excellent store for all natural insulation products is Ecological Building Systems (**www.ecologicalbuildingsystems.co.uk**).

A ground-breaking eco-development in Cornwall is the Trelowarren estate of eco-timeshare/self-catering homes (**www.trelowarren.com**). These houses are built from all-natural materials, and timber frames are used with a void of 300 ml and recycled newspaper insulation, which gives a high thermal mass. If you're lucky enough to be contemplating a new build, go and have a look, or just have a wonderful week's holiday.

And while we're on insulation, make sure your hot water pipes are lagged. I've found that almost anything goes, even old towels and blankets – not particularly eco, apart from the energy-saving, but as you know, I love an old-style simple solution.

LIGHTING

Energy-saving bulbs (CFLs)

We've known about energy-saving light bulbs for years now, and there is much information available on how important they are in the saving energy cause, compared to regular incandescent light bulbs, which waste energy by giving off heat.

I read some interesting research that claimed that there are over 600 million light sockets in the UK, and on average 12 per cent of a household's electricity bill, is due to lights. We're told that if we all used energy-saving light bulbs

'The ultimate "computer", our own brain, uses only ten watts of power – one-tenth the energy consumed by a 100-watt bulb.' Paul Valéry, poet, critic

we could save enough electricity to close down two power stations (not sure where the workforce would be re-employed), but perhaps a more interesting fact is that Philip Selwood of the Energy Saving Trust reckons that if everyone in the UK installed just three energy-saving light bulbs we would save enough energy to power the UK's street lighting for a year. Now that's impressive!

But are they really as green as we'd like to think? Firstly, they are more costly and use more energy to create than standard bulbs when you take into account the complete manufacture, packaging and distribution process. In use, I would expect the extra cost of a bulb to be paid off in six months (though interestingly, not a large percentage of my energy savers seem to last more than six months). However, according to the US Department of Energy, turning them on and off frequently appears to shorten their life. A 1998 study of electronically ballasted CFLs found in the case of a five-minute switch on/off cycle, the lifespan of a CFL can be reduced by up to 85 per cent, bringing their lifespan back on a par with that of incandescent bulbs.

Most importantly, they contain mercury, currently the World Health Organisation's number one environmental poison, now banned by the EU from landfill sites. I must confess that before I realised this I simply chucked dead ones in the bin. I checked the packaging recently on several types. Two do not mention safe disposal at all, one has a tiny diagram of a bin with a cross through it, and another, the Ecobulb, has an inscription on the actual bulb reading 'Contains mercury – dispose according to local, state or federal laws'. Ah, helpful, then. What on earth happens if we break one by accident? Presumably we need to call in the cavalry. I rang my local council and was told to just wrap it up and put it in the bin, or, if you want to recycle, check with your local recycling centre. I pointed out that I thought the bulbs contained mercury, and 'Isn't that hazardous waste?', to which their reply was that they didn't have any information about that, but perhaps they could find out and call me back.

I then called Waste Aware, who quoted a few lines at me from their website and, in answer to the question 'Is it imperative that I take the light bulbs to a recycling centre?', said, 'Well, obviously you can put anything you want to in the regular bin' (incorrect answer, I think you'll find), and when I asked what to do in the case of one being broken the answer given was 'Put all the bits into a bag and take to the recycling centre' as before. I then rang three UK websites that sell energy-saving light bulbs and asked what I should do if one is accidentally broken. It was clear none were aware of any potential danger, and all three suggested that I simply put the remains into a bag and either take to the recycling centre (if still relatively in one piece) or just 'put it in the bin'.

In truth, energy-saving light bulbs are what is classed as 'hazardous waste'. One fluorescent light tube can contain enough mercury to contaminate 30,000 litres of drinking water, and incidentally I was under the impression that there were fines of thousands of pounds in place for the incorrect disposal of hazardous waste. Confusion reigns!

In the United States they are a little further ahead and give clear guidelines for disposal. They advise: do not vacuum up; open the windows for

15 minutes; using rubber gloves, scoop up the broken bits with cardboard and then use duct tape to pick up any remaining bits; and place in a sealed bag before taking to a recycling centre, where it will then be subject to 'hazardous waste' laws. Hang on, I thought the point of these light bulbs was to be green! When buying CFLs for The Garrack Hotel in Cornwall, the owner noticed that the invoice contained a three-pound surcharge to 'WEE' (see Recycling, page 52). He intends to collect them as they stop working and take them all back to the supplier for recycling – it will be interesting to see what's in place for the surcharge paid.

It therefore remains a worry for me that the current stance on CFLs is that they are regarded as the saviours of the green cause, and we're left with the slightly unreassuring fact that 600 million of these little mercury bombs could be adorning our houses in years to come – and in a classic bit of knee-jerk politics, they could become virtually compulsory.

Also, some people are incandescent with rage, because the light isn't that nice and CFLs aren't appropriate in every interior space. They won't always do the job of creating that feel you need, and that's an important part of a healthy home too. Recent reports have linked CFLs with increased migraines in sufferers. (Remember those reports of workers suffering depression and stress in offices lit by fluorescent lights in the 1970/80s?) That said, in their defence, the technology is changing all the time, and I'm sure that even as we speak, designers and manufacturers are developing and introducing many improvements to counteract all these shortcomings.

Another interesting by-product of the boom in energy-saving bulbs is that they emit less heat, so technically the demands on central heating could be greater. Not such a mad point, really. It's possible that a fifth of the claimed savings in carbon might be lost because of the increased need to heat the house in winter. My friend Jennifer says, 'My three 100-watt spot lights in my kitchen raise the temperature along the worktops, which is just where I need it, by up to 2°C, which allows me to set the background heating to the kitchen at 18°C.'

In any case we don't have an option; really we're stuck with them. But the future could be light-emitting diodes (LEDs), like the coloured ones that mean your TV is on standby. These don't contain any hazardous materials, but they are expensive and currently not available to replace all our household bulbs. At the time of going to print (things are changing fast) LEDs can only replace a 20-watt halogen bulb, but they're great for a nice intimate lounge area. The only worry is that they could go the same way as the no-sharpen razor or 'ladderless' tights – what company will want to manufacture a product that will need replacing only every ten years? Interestingly traffic lights now use LEDs in some areas. For more on LEDs and solar-powered lights, see page 63.

Leaving lights on when they aren't needed can account for 10–15 per cent extra energy use and I must confess I'm horribly guilty of this. If you've come to rely on leaving lights on as security so that would-be burglars will assume you're at home, invest instead in some security timers that switch lamps and radios on and off randomly. Anyone 'casing your joint' is more likely to think you're at home if there's no real pattern to it. It goes without saying: turn lights off. A religious dedication to 'switching off when not in use' can make an even better saving than changing to CFLs. I know people who are much more lax about turning off now they're using energy savers – back to square one!

ENERGY-SAVING ON APPLIANCES

I still get a shock when I get my electricity bill and always welcome ways to reduce it. The difficulty can be working out where to make the savings. One gadget that helps is The Owl, a device that clips on to the household electrical supply and monitors the amount of wasted electricity. It also tells you the cost and the CO2 emissions. It costs about £50, so it's not cheap, but over a couple of years you'll save far more than that in theory, and again it's a great tool for making children aware that energy has a price. It's sold in B&Q and from www.ethicalsuperstore.co.uk.

You know the advice: switch all electrical appliances off at the wall when not in use (no standbys, please), not only to save energy but to reduce EMFs, which will still be emitting from cables even when appliances are switched off (see page 136). In truth it's a hassle, though, isn't it? Fortunately there are a few gadgets to help us now. If you have more than one item of electrical equipment, there's the Powersafer Multi AV power-saving device for approximately £25 from www.green warehouse.co.uk You plug it into the mains and then you can plug up to five units – DVD, hi-fi, etc. into it – and then when you switch them off using the remote control, the power saver will cut the electricity supply until you switch back on.

Of course you don't want to be re-booting your computer every hour, but you can now get a Oneclick 'Intelliplug' or intelligent panel (see www.oneclick power.com), which eliminates the excessive standby use by automatically cutting off power to all the peripheral appliances such as monitor, printer and scanner, which don't need to be left on while your computer is in standby mode. The Oneclick costs around £30 or £17 for the Intelliplug and uses only 0.6 watts when in off mode, so the theory is it should save you on average 35 watts an hour.

There's also the Bye Bye Standby (from www.eco hamster.co.uk), which is a clever combination of smart sockets and remote control that allows you to cut power to any appliance consuming energy in standby mode with the touch of a button on the remote control.

Cutting power to your appliances rather than leaving them on standby is likely to cut up to £40 from the average bill each year.

Having recommended all the above products, I must say I'm inclined to err on the side of reducing the amount of electronic gadgetry and some of the radio frequency devices that work through walls, which I'd personally rather avoid (see page 134), so if you're fit and able, a really old-style tip is to get into a habit of just bending down to flick a switch!

Fridge-freezers are expensive to run and one way of reducing the cost by 20 per cent is to fit a Savaplug. This replaces the existing plug and works on a thermostat basis; once the motor is running, the Savaplug reduces the flow of electricity to match the actual requirement, and you can see a red light glowing that shows savings are being made. It's not suitable for all types of fridge-freezers, so you'll need to do some research to check if it's of any use to you. It costs around £22. It's one of those gadgets that can take a couple of years to pay for itself, but it does come with a ten-year guarantee.

For more on responsible energy use, see page 67 [Renewable energy].

SOLAR ENERGY

There are so many new developments in this area, and the gradual demise of the battery mountain can only be good news. Select Solar (www.selectsolar.co.uk) makes a big range of solar gadgets and gizmos from torches to toys, which are a great way to get into the whole concept of solar, especially for children. I get these little gizmos for them so that hopefully by the time they're paying their own energy bills, the idea of eco power alternatives will be second nature. You can even get a kit to make a solar-powered wooden toy windmill, at around £15 from www.the-green-apple.co.uk. Select Solar also sell a great range of chargers for your phone and laptop, as do Ethical Superstore (www.ethical.superstore.com), who do the excellent Freeloader – no, not a hungry musician who expects to crash out on your floor but a solar-powered charger for just about everything.

Big solar

Instead of paying for electricity, why not make it yourself? Some day all houses will be equipped with self-generating supplies, but for now, it's a retro fit. There are many options to look at, and the technology is improving all the time. The ones we mostly see on many rooftops are photovoltaic (PV) panels, which work off sunlight, or even just 'light' on a cloudy day. Okay for enhancing an existing supply, but it's still at the moment quite a big investment for the power you get. But if you're keen to go down this route, you don't have to dive in at the deep end and at websites such as **www.solarcentury.co.uk** you can scan through many options to see what fits your budget. It's also possible to get government grants for such projects, though there are finite resources that can be allocated.

The Energy Saving Trust has lots of advice and help lines. Call your local advice centre on 0800 512 012 or see **www.est.org.uk**.

Solar heating

Solar heating comes in the form of add-on systems that can give you more than half of your domestic hot water, and they seem a better bet than photovoltaic (PV) panels. They use 'thermal' solar panels, which look pretty similar to PVs, but they heat your water rather than give you electricity. They can be integrated into most existing systems, and are pretty maintenance-free. A good concept, and it would probably be my system of choice. Again you may be able to get a grant if you install one, on average around 30 per cent of the cost. Here's an account of a friend of mine in Cornwall, Sally Pryner, who had a system installed.

We decided to get a solar hot-water heating system when an elderly friend died and I inherited some money. We couldn't think of a finer way to remember him, really – every time the sun shines!

We used Cornish company Celtic Solar Limited (www.celticsolar.co.uk).

The total cost of the installation was £2,986 and we got a government 'clearskies grant' (given in some areas for installing solar panels) of £500 off that. It was installed in September 2004 and the other day I looked at the ticker they installed to measure how many hours of solar hot water we have harvested (three years on) and it was at 4,700 hours. That impressed me anyway!

Because our house is so small, we could not have as much storage for the hot water tank as we wanted, but got the largest cylinder we could to fit into the smallest space possible. The tank has two coils inside instead of the usual one, so that the solar system has access to the lower coil, and the immersion and boiler to the top one.

The solar panel is a very simple horizontal 'flat plate' collection system, which sits on top of our roof. A sensor detects when the sun is shining enough to start up and then the pump starts, making a very quiet ticking noise, which is always quite reassuring. There is a small photovoltaic plate (generating electricity from the sun) to power the pump that takes hot water from the pipes inside the panel to our storage tank, where it stays hot for 48 hours. From the cylinder to our taps it works in the same way as any other hot water heating system, sending it to our bath and sinks. It is a shame we didn't have downstairs space for the hot water tank because if we did, we'd have been able to run a small radiator for the run-off (water gets incredibly hot – especially as we took the regulator out of our system to ensure our boiler didn't just override any heat produced by the sun). The more plates and storage you have, the more you can run off it (e.g. whole central heating systems).

The only downside to the solar system is needing to 'run off' hot water on a very hot day and, occasionally, when you could really do with it, you don't have enough. But generally, now there are children in the house and they never refuse a bath – we don't have to run off much and, also, if we keep an eye on the weather, we know when not to run off the hot and save it for the next couple of days if it looks like being a bit cold and dark.

I couldn't have chosen a better way to spend an inheritance (I suppose if it was masses of money we'd have gone one step further to a wind turbine!). We love the fact that we are less reliant upon electricity and fossil fuels now, and we have a great landmark if people are trying to find our house. Mind you, it's a pity we can't say we're the tenth solar panel on the street instead of the only one.

OTHER WAYS TO ENHANCE A HEATING SYSTEM

Air source heat pumps attach on the side of a building and look a bit like air con units. They take energy from the outside air and raise it to a higher temperature. They can generate up to four times the power they use. Quite a good option costwise, although they probably work best in countries that don't have very cold winters, and they can be noisy.

Similarly ground source heat pumps use a below-ground 'loop' to extract and transfer energy. Though they are very efficient, there's a fair bit of installation costs and digging up of your garden. Both pumps use similar technology to that of your regular fridge.

WIND TURBINES

'Micro' turbines can be fitted rather like TV aerials to your chimneystack, and are now on sale at some of the big DIY stores. At best they will generate a few hundred watts on a windy day, enough to run a bunch of energy-efficient light bulbs. Other days you'll be lucky to light one bulb for a few hours, so you'd have to be pretty dedicated to reducing your CO2 emissions with these, as it could take you more than ten years to make up the installation costs – if you're lucky, some might say.

The bigger 'mini' turbines are more efficient, but you can get into eyesore and noise-level issues in urban areas. Some people, though, think they're beautiful (see the account below). I know someone who couldn't get planning permission so installed one of these on a trailer, which turns it into a legal 'movable feast'.

At the current level of technology and cost, wind power in a domestic situation is possibly more about making an eco statement, albeit a very worthy one, than making a real saving. There are people willing to take the plunge, and thanks to them this can only encourage further technological developments and improvements. I think I'm going to leave it for a few years before delving more. For more information, go to **www.reuk.co.uk**, the website of Renewable Energy UK..

> *'Who has seen the wind? Neither you nor I but when the trees bow down their heads, the wind is passing by.'* Christina Rossetti

Here's an account by Harvey Davis, the husband of one of my website forum members, Nyree Davis.

Why we bought the wind turbine:
- *To reduce our dependence on expensive, bought-in energy*
- *To make more of our local wind resource.*
- *We love wind turbines and it looks beautiful spinning gracefully on the hill behind our house – kind of like a dynamic sculpture!*

Costs:
Ground works and trenching: £3,000. Our turbine is situated about 200 metres |from our house, so there was a lot of trench to dig for the cable. Turbine supply and install: £17,500. We used Segen Ltd (www.segen.co.uk), which is the sole UK distributor of Iskra turbines, which are made in the UK.

We received a grant of £5,000 from the Energy Saving Trust, making the total cost about £15,000. The whole process took about six months.

Segen was a great company to deal with. They are installing about two turbines a week in the UK at the moment. They organise open days where you can visit homes that have installed one of their turbines, which we did, and it was a really useful process to see the real thing in situ and get the homeowner's opinions.

How it works:
The turbine stands on a hill behind our house on a 36-foot-high, freestanding steel mast. It is grid-connected. We have two 'inverters', which ensure a seamless, uninterrupted supply of electricity, and we have never needed to touch the system. We also have two electricity meters, one for normal electricity and one for the turbine.

The turbine can produce a maximum power of 5,300 watts (5.3 kw). The average kettle requires about 3,000 watts (3 kw).

The supply from the turbine is variable, as is our household demand for power. Therefore, whether we are taking power from the turbine or from the grid is constantly changing, depending on the wind speed and which appliances are being used in the house. Both meters have a flashing red light that indicates a flow of power. If both meters are flashing, then you know that the turbine is producing power but the household's demand is higher, so it is drawing from the turbine and the grid at the same time. On a fairly windy day, the turbine could be generating up to 5,300 watts as the wind gusts and maybe only 200 watts in between gusts. If there is nobody at home, then during gusts the turbine will generate more power than the house requires and the excess flows on to the grid.

On more than a few occasions on windy days, I've put the kettle or a fan heater on and watched what happens to the meters. It can get quite obsessive. (Nyree thinks I'm a bit sad and should try and get out more!) Over the first four months we generated 655 units of electricity.

One important point is that during a power cut we cannot use power from the turbine. The turbine needs the connection to the grid to fill in the gaps between gusts of wind and to stabilise the voltage. The system automatically disconnects the turbine from the grid during a power cut so that engineers can safely work on the fault.

RENEWABLE ENERGY SUPPLIERS

I must confess that until I made myself look into this in the name of research I was thoroughly daunted by the whole idea of switching to a green energy supplier. We've all had people with clipboards accosting us in the high street advising us to change our supplier to save money, and some of us have changed only to find that the new company's tariff changes and we might as well have stayed put. At one time it was easy and there was just one supplier for gas and one for electricity, but now there is a bewildering array of service providers we can choose from.

But what is 'green energy' or renewable energy? Well, simply that which comes from renewable sources such as wind and water, and doesn't directly result in by-products. Because it limits waste, its impact on the environment is far lighter than that of regular energy.

The important thing to remember is there is no change in the actual power you use. A proportion of what you pay is matched to units of electricity to be fed into the national grid from renewable sources. Good Energy Ltd (**www.good-energy.co.uk**) pledges to match 100 per cent of the units of electricity you buy from them with an equal amount from renewable sources; so for

example for every unit of electricity you buy from them they will supply the national grid with a unit that has been generated from a source such as wind, the sun or water.

There are lots of suppliers offering green energy now and you'll be pleased to know it's well regulated. Some also offer incentives to homeowners to generate their own power, and pay them for their achievements.

Friends of the Earth recommend certain green suppliers and give reasons for their selections at **www.foe.co.uk**.

Ever the cynic, though, I must voice my concern that some companies offering 'green tariffs' charge more and are directly using customers' money (and charging us for the privilege) to invest in renewables, which I wonder if they should have been doing under new and coming guidelines or legislation anyway.

There's excellent advice at **www.energysavingsecrets.co.uk**, **www.greenhelpline.com** and **www.downwithco2.co.uk**.

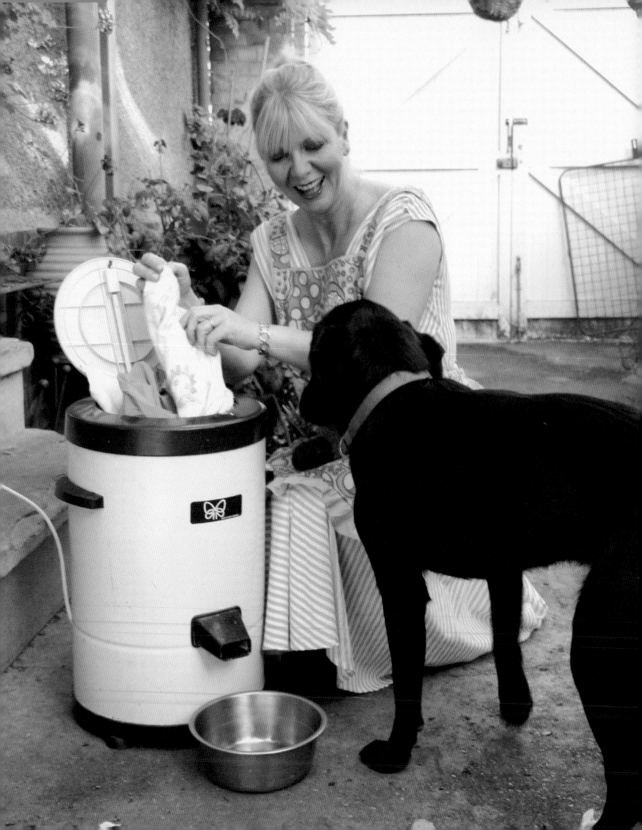

6 Household appliances

'By his very success in inventing labour-saving devices, modern man has manufactured an abyss of boredom that only the privileged classes in earlier civilisations have ever fathomed.'

Lewis Mumford, writer

There are of course some gadgets available now to help reduce the energy usage of many of our household appliances, but how do we ensure that our 'white goods' are 'green' and that other basic kitchen and household appliances are efficient and eco-friendly? For appliances generally, see the website of the Energy Savings Trust, **www.est.org.uk**, which has a database of the electrical appliances that are the most energy-efficient. Here are some thoughts on individual appliances.

COOKERS

As I write this, I'm trying to decide quite what to do. We have a big double stainless-steel range electric oven with a gas hob, but it's very elderly and the seals are less than ideal now. I know that energy is being wasted, so it's a difficult decision whether to get it repaired –

new seals and an overhaul – or buy a new one.

As a rule, gas hobs and ovens tend to be more efficient, and personally I can't stand electric hobs. Ceramic hobs with halogen elements seem difficult to control for me but rate fairly well for efficiency. Fan-assisted electric ovens use heat up more quickly, saving time and power overall; and there are now induction hobs, which are said to be 82 per cent efficient. I have a few friends with huge Agas in their homely kitchen, and while I don't think it's fair to call them 'energy-efficient' an Aga does make the kitchen beautifully warm, so reducing central heating bills for several months of the year, so if you have one already don't beat yourself up, and just enjoy.

For true innovation, have a look at the Centre for Sustainable Futures' website, **www.csf.plymouth.ac.uk**. They offer a course where you can 'Learn to build a super-efficient wood-fuelled Rocket Stove and make a small portable stove to take home with you', ideal for outside use and fine for indoors so long as it's well ventilated. Maybe for a rainy day!

MICROWAVE OVENS

It's true that they use less energy than conventional ovens, but at what cost? Personally I detest microwave ovens and never use one. I think they contribute to the increase in packaging by encouraging people to eat ready meals, and I don't like what they do to the food, changing its molecular structure. If you are going to use one, use it for a 'quick fix' – defrosting, reheating, etc. – but remember that potatoes will need almost as long to cook in the microwave as boiling on the hob, and the taste is not comparable.

VACUUM CLEANERS

In terms of health I'd say opt for one with a HEPA filter, particularly if you have dust allergies, respiratory problems or asthma, or of course pets that leave hairs behind. The Miele Dog and Cat is excellent. There are models with 'high-efficiency filters' that minimise the re-emission of dust, such as Medivac (www.medivac.co.uk).

Bagless vacuum cleaners probably use fewer resources, and therefore have less environmental impact, but be wary when you empty the machine, as the dust particles could be flying around as they hit the dustbin. For more info on allergies, see www.healthy-house.co.uk.

WASHING MACHINES

Sadly I'm too imperfect to want to go back to the 1950s on this one. I absolutely wouldn't want to be constantly hand-washing or using a copper and a mangle. However, washing machines use a massive amount of energy and waste a huge amount of water, so it's good to try to reduce our usage of both.

Eco laundry products will help: using laundry balls or soapnuts (see page 23) will do away with the need for pre-wash or rinse cycles. Of course we can do the obvious by making sure we always wash only a full load and use the economy cycle. Temperatures are important too. As we have seen, most loads can be done at 30°C, which is now the recommended temperature. But what are the most efficient brands of washing machine?

Look for an A-rated machine such as the Miele W1714.

There are some great developments from LG (www.uk.lge.com), who make the Steam Direct Drive. The bad news is that it's around £800, but it washes a huge load (a whopping four cubic feet), so it's great for big families, and it's wonderfully energy-saving, as it uses steam, which means it actually uses about 35 per cent less water than regular machines of a similar size, and 20 per cent less electricity. The really interesting bit is that it also does away with the need for ironing, as the steam leaves the laundry 'wrinkle free' (wish I could get one for my face!), and the manufacturers claim there's no need for detergents either. Hopefully we'll see some of those innovations incorporated into cheaper models in the future.

Electrolux have given a green design award to the E-wash, which is half the size of conventional machines and designed to work with soapnuts, making sure they're added to the cycle at the right time. I'm not sure that's necessary, unless the price is really competitive, as in my experience, soapnuts work with all machines.

If you are replacing your washing machine look for one with energy efficient A or an AA rating and an 'economy' option. Also ask the retailer to come and get your old one. You can get more info on energy efficiency from www.defra.gov.uk/environment or call 0800 512012.To find an ethical brand, go to www.gooshing.co.uk.

TUMBLE AND SPIN DRYERS

Tumblers are very eco-unfriendly, but you can slash their use by 75 per cent by spending about £15 in a junk shop on an old-style top-loading spin dryer – you know, the kind your mum used to have (see page 27).

If you do want to 'tumble' invest in an energy efficient machine. Find an A rated appliance using 2.52KH such as the AEG T59800.

FRIDGES AND FREEZERS

A veritable minefield, this one. Old-style domestic fridge-freezers that use powerful greenhouse gas refrigerants (CFCs and HFCs) are a great concern for green campaigners. Fortunately, new fridges no longer use them, mostly using HC (hydrocarbon) refrigerants instead, which have no impact on the ozone layer. R600, a hydrocarbon coolant, which is labelled CFC- and HFC-free, is apparently more efficient than CFCs and has lower global warming potential.

Interestingly you could save money over time, and certainly do your bit for the planet, by investing in a new fridge if yours is not energy-efficient. Avoid frost-free ones because they never 'let up' and opt for an energy rating of A++. The EU also awards 'eco labels' to energy-efficient models if they're manufactured with minimal environmental impact.

Defrosting freezers regularly is a complete pain but the only way to safeguard their efficiency. My trusted larder fridge, only around three years old, broke down and I was convinced I'd have to replace it, but I got a tip off from a fridge-freezer engineer who said, 'Take off the panel right at the back of the fridge (inside) and there you'll probably find a solid block of ice.' Well, I got DH (darling husband) on the job and sure enough it was very fiddly, but after some tugging he pulled away a solid sheet of ice, like a large opaque mirror. The fridge has been fine ever since.

When choosing a freezer, opt for an upright rather than a chest variety, unless you have a big family, and try to keep it filled to capacity (or at least with scrunched-up newspaper in the gaps) as this uses less electricity.

DISHWASHERS

I must confess that with a big family, I can't live without a dishwasher, but before you berate me and tell me to go back to regular washing up, remember that some people can actually use more water over the course of the day by washing up three or four times and leaving the tap running to rinse the dishes.

Imperfectly natural home Q&A

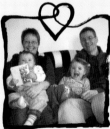

Donna Stephenson

Describe your home
Four-bedrooms, detached, garage and large, barren garden.

Who lives here?
Five people, a cat and 11 tropical fish.

How would you describe your interior 'style' and furnishings? Probably comfortable, warm and mostly modern would sum us up best.

What does your home mean to you?
Somewhere comfortable and secure to bring up my family.

Have you attempted any eco DIY or modifications for a greener home? E.g. solar panels, eco paints, wind turbines etc. Was it worth it financially? Have replaced all light bulbs with low-energy ones, have two composters and a green cone. Am considering a wind turbine and/or ground source heat pump.

How would your home rate for energy-efficiency? What have you done to reduce energy usage? When you buy new appliances do you consider the energy efficiency? I would say my house is reasonably energy-efficient as it is very well insulated. As mentioned above, I've replaced all my bulbs with energy-efficient ones. Try to use minimal heating (not easy in the north of Scotland) and not use standby on things. I do consider energy-efficiency of new appliances when buying them.

What ideas do you have for water saving?
None really, as it isn't an issue where I live. We have more than enough water for our island.

How 'eco' is your furniture, floorings and furnishings? I only buy furniture and floorings when they really are worn out and buy second-hand wherever possible, they are quite 'eco' from that point of view.

What cleaning/laundry/stain-removing products do you use? For laundry I mostly use Ecover non-bio liquid with either vanish soap or Ecover stain remover. I do have a box of bio powder for occasional use. However, it gets more use as a general stain remover on carpets when potty training etc. Household cleaning is mostly achieved with bicarb of soda, vinegar, lemon juice, microfibre cloths and elbow grease, although I confess to bleaching the loos once a week.

If you could buy any one 'eco' gadget or item for your home inside or out what would it be? Ground-source heat pump for heating the house.

What kind of cookware do you use? Non-stick/cast iron? I have one non-stick pan, the rest are steel.

What's your best tip for getting your fridge and larder stocked with healthy food? Fruit, veggies and fresh fish come from the mobile shop that comes round weekly. I get an organic veg box from a local grower in season but the season here only lasts a couple of months. The rest of my groceries come from the local supermarket supplemented by a few bits and pieces from the health-food shop and deli.

What about composting? We compost all fruit, veggie peels and coffee grounds along with some paper. Have two composters and a green cone.

What do you regularly recycle? Everything. There is no doorstep collection here so we load up the estate car and go to the dump about once a month, which is about a mile away.

If you have a garden, what are your eco tips? I do have a garden but don't have any eco tips as I'm still getting to grips with it.

Have you ever considered 'Feng Shui' for your home? No, I think Feng Shui is a way of parting daft folks from their money.

What are your views on the possible dangers of electro 'smog'/wifi/emfs etc.? Have you taken any protective measures for your family? Undecided on this but don't have wifi etc. anyway so it's not an issue. Neighbours are far enough away not to have too many worries.

Do you know your carbon footprint and do you care about it? (Be honest!) I don't know my carbon footprint but it does worry me. As we live on a small island, everything is shipped or even air-freighted in (mostly shipped though) and all our waste is shipped out (though it does go to a neighbouring island to be incinerated to heat public buildings). I think because of where we live our footprint is quite high even when trying to consume the minimum.

How green are you – lime/olive? Probably mid-green.

Do you have an imperfectly natural guilty secret? As mentioned – bleaching the lavvies weekly!

What would your dream home be like? Well insulated, full of light and low energy use. Probably heated by ground source heat-pump. I'd like it to sit well in its surroundings and have lots of trees around and a fab view.

What are your top three tips for a naturally healthy home? 1. Don't buy things you don't need. 2. Bicarb and lemons clean most things. 3. Draw the curtains at dusk on colder nights – it makes a huge difference to the amount of heat lost.

7 Natural remedies

Common ailments affect us all from time to time, but how can we treat the symptoms without resorting to pharmaceutical products? Well, that one's easy: nature has actually provided us with all we need, and sometimes being old-style really is the best. Before you head off to the chemist to treat a cold, tummy bug or headache, stop and see what's in your kitchen cupboards or fridge and keep a 'natural medicine cabinet'. . .

Please bear in mind all the remedies below are suggestions only and if symptoms persist, always consult your practitioner.

For extensive information on holistic dentistry, alternative therapies and treatments, including homeopathy, exercise, better eyesight without glasses and how our mental and spiritual state affects our health, please refer to *Imperfectly Natural Woman*. For tips on natural remedies for babies and young children, see *Imperfectly Natural Baby and Toddler*.

It's worth investing in a homeopathic kit that comes with a guide on how to self-prescribe. There are excellent kits at **www.ainsworths.com** and **www.helios.com**. A really good 'bible' is the *Complete Guide to Homeopathy* by Miranda Castro.

Treat yourself to a beautifully designed chart from **www.lemonburst.co.uk** to remind you what to reach for in the heat of the ailment.

BITES AND STINGS

For nettle stings, reach for dock leaves (usually found growing in the vicinity of the nettles), and for wasp stings reach for the vinegar (any will do). For a bee sting, use bicarbonate of soda mixed with water or a little milk. You can now buy Instant Relief, an excellent spray containing healing helichrysum, from **www.sensitive skincareco.com**. The homeopathic remedy apis works brilliantly if you take it as soon as you've been bitten. **www.helios.com**

If you feel you go through a period of getting more than your fair share of bites, one interesting theory is that you may be lacking in B vitamins, so consider taking a supplement for a while.

BRUISES

It's become almost as common as aspirin: arnica is fantastic for bruising (and shock). Use arnica cream, and if the bruising is severe, take a pillule of Arnica 30. Most high-street chemists sell it now.

Arnica is also useful for more serious situations, such as when you are about to have an operation: take Arnica 200 for a few days before the op and continue again during the recovery period.

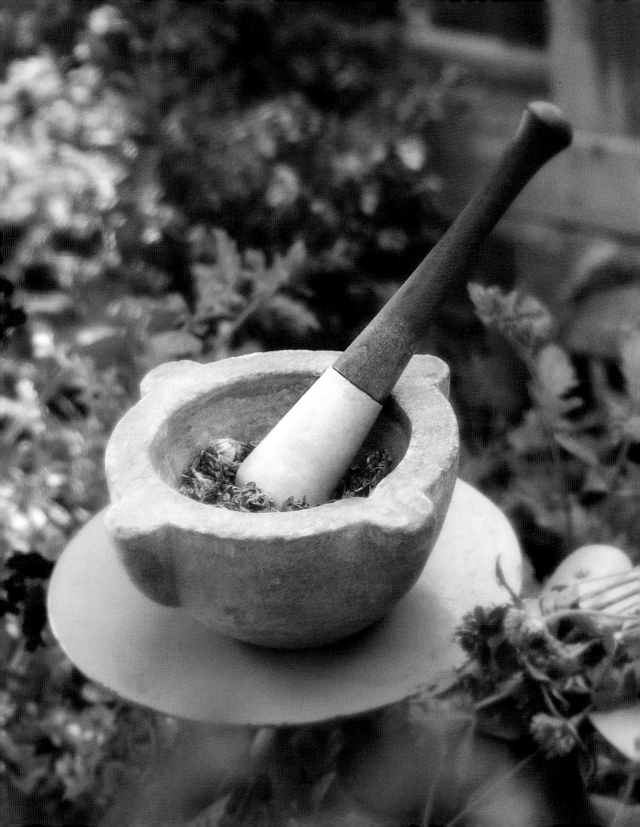

If the bruise is inflamed, apply a cold vinegar compress or use witch hazel on a pad of cotton wool.

MILD BURNS AND SCALDS

For a minor burn or scald, snip an aloe vera plant and use the juice (not great for the plant, I know) or apply neat lavender oil, which works incredibly quickly.

COLDS AND FLU

During winter, forget stocking up your medicine cabinet with commercial medicines for coughs, colds, etc., and remember old-fashioned remedies like honey and lemon in hot water. Many respiratory problems can be cured with steam: just fill a bowl with boiled water, add a drop of tea tree or eucalyptus oil to the water, put a towel over your head and steam away. This is also a great way to help children with respiratory problems. Sit with them to keep them safe under a big blanket or towel and play tents, or you can get the bathroom all steamy and add some eucalyptus oil to the water.

At bathtime, add a cupful of Epsom salts |to the water or better still Himalayan salt, which has wonderfully healing and detoxifying properties (you can also use it directly on your food or for healthy cooking too) – go to www.saltshack.co.uk or www.amazinghealth.co.uk.

Echinacea has been up and down in the media, some studies saying it's effective, others claiming it has no benefit. Echinacea purpurea or purple coneflower is the full name of the herb, and I'm a big believer in its healing properties and immune-boosting powers. I suggest using it as soon as you feel the first signs of a cold or sore throat, or if you're around other people who are suffering, combine it with high doses of vitamin C for a few days and you should get over the cold more quickly.

Sage is also excellent for sore throats and the pioneers of echinacea, Bioforce, now make an excellent Echinacea Throat Spray, which contains sage too. Available in most health stores or from www.avogel.co.uk.

Viridian (www.viridian.co.uk) do an excellent Cold Season pack.

As a vegetarian I don't eat chicken soup, but I'm assured by very wise people that it really is therapeutic in many ways. Make sure you buy an organic chicken.

Manuka honey is antibacterial and soothing (see www.manukahoney.co.uk). Take it by the spoonful (with a little crushed garlic it's even more powerful) or spread it on rye toast. The higher the Unique Manuka Factor (UMF) activity rating, the better (this refers to the live 'activity' grade of the honey.). Ginger is fantastic for colds too; keep fresh ginger in the freezer and then just pop a grated spoonful or two into a pan with hot water and lemon, simmer it, strain and sip throughout the day.

Propolis is excellent; you can buy Propolis lozenges that are really soothing for a sore throat from health food shops.

MINOR CUTS

Honey is an all-round healer that can be applied to wounds too. Manuka honey (see above) is good for cuts as it's antibacterial. Look for a high 'activity' rating of +16 or more if you can afford it, but any honey will do the job.

Use calendula cream, hypercal cream or the excellent Neem Antibacterial Wound Cream, from www.junglesale.com.

Z-Gel (available from www.mint-elabs.com) is an all-purpose natural gel that soothes minor cuts and bruises, itchy or irritated skin, insect stings and sunburn. It's safe enough to be used even in the mouth.

CYSTITIS AND THRUSH

Avoid dairy and sugars for a few days, take a good probiotic and head for your bed with a hot water bottle! Drink copious amounts of water and, if you can get it, unsweetened cranberry juice. Make your own lemon barley water too, but use a natural sweetener such as organic agave nectar (from the Mexican agave plant) or manuka honey rather than sugar. Aloe vera gel can help too.

EARACHE

Drop a couple of drops of warmed olive oil into the ear. Try massaging a couple of drops of lavender or chamomile oil, in a base oil such as jojoba oil, gently around the ear.

FEELING BLUE

Obviously if you're clinically depressed it's imperative that you seek professional help, but for those winter blues there's a fair bit you can do to lift your spirits. Firstly go for a walk in the fresh air. Studies show that walking outdoors every single day greatly helps anxiety and depression. If you can afford one, invest in a light therapy box: you don't have to be actually suffering from seasonal affective disorder (SAD) to feel the benefit on winter afternoons (see page 112).

Vitamin B has a big role to play in the relief of stress and anxiety, so make sure you're taking them. So, too, do the vital omega 3s (see page 37). Take a good-quality blend of oil such as Udo's Choice, available in good health shops, or one of the less heavy versions such as Cool Oil, a mix of omega 3, 6 and 9, available in supermarkets or from www.groovy food.co.uk, and eat nuts and seeds and consider trying health kinesiology to determine any deficiencies (www.hk4health.co.uk).

FIBROMYALGIA, ARTHRITIC PAIN AND MUSCLE PAIN

These conditions must of course be checked by a medical doctor but often there are things you can do to help yourself alongside conventional treatments. MSM (methylsulphonylmethane) supplements from www.highernature.com are said to be very good at relieving symptoms. Recently a friend with fairly serious fibromyalgia has found that her symptoms are greatly relieved and she is now sleeping well because of the amazing benefits of drinking cherry juice – Montmorency cherries to be exact. It's been claimed it cures gout (bit late for Henry VIII) and helps arthritis. It's available from www.cherryactive.co.uk, and is also available in capsule form if you don't want to drink it. It also tastes great as a cordial or as a tea.

The Bowen technique is a non-invasive treatment that I highly recommend for any types of muscle pain. See my *Imperfectly Natural Woman* and check www.thebowen technique.com.

I also recommend magnetic therapy for many ailments, including pains and inflammation. There's lots of info in my first two books, on page 79 and at www.ecoflow.com.

HEADACHES AND INFLAMMATIONS

Feverfew is very quick acting for pain relief. It's also anti-inflammatory. You can take it tablet form and you can make a tea by adding boiling water to the capsule's contents. Buy it from health food shops but it's not advised if you're pregnant. Tiger balm is soothing rubbed along the temples. Avoid the type with a paraffin base and find a natural one that contains coconut oil or beeswax. Try the Head Ease Balm from www.livingnature.co.uk (or if you're feeling creative, try making your own – www.care2.com has some recipes). Remember, too, to drink lots of water to get rid of a headache quickly.

You can also use the natural version of aspirin, white willow, available in capsules as Willow Complex from www.revital.co.uk. Hippocrates mentioned around 400 BC that decoctions of willow bark are effective in cases of inflammation of the joints, pain and fever.

INSOMNIA

See page 113 for how to create the perfect environment for sleep and always consider what you eat before bedtime. Bananas, lettuce and turkey are all sleep-inducing foods but avoid alcohol and coffee for obvious reasons.

Drink chamomile tea, and for tired eyes

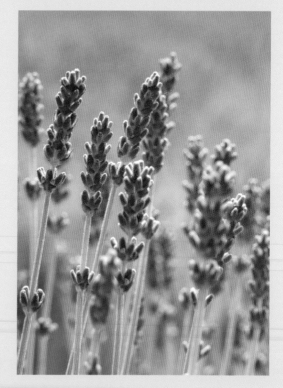

relax with chamomile tea bags over your eyes (once cooled, of course!). You can also get The Chillow, a personal cooling pad that contains water but doesn't need to be refrigerated. Great for anyone who suffers from night sweats. www.eoco.org.uk

Lavender oil can be very effective. Put some directly on to your pillow or put a few drops into an aromatherapy burner. Use the Herb Sacks from www.dreamacres.co.uk and the excellent Sleep Easy essence from www.indigoessences.com.

Valerian, melissa and lemon balm are known to promote sleep. You can buy capsules from MedicHerb (www.medicherb.co.uk).

IRRITABLE BOWEL

If your symptoms persist, always seek help, but as a precautionary measure make sure you take a good probiotic to aid digestion. You can eat natural live yoghurt but avoid probiotic drinks that can contain sugars. If you take capsules, bear in mind you should store them in the fridge. If you prefer probiotic powder, a really easy way to take it is in a fresh smoothie along with hemp or flax oil from good supermarkets or health shops and your favourite fruits and yoghurt.

Keep the homeopathic remedy nux vomica to hand: it's good for digestive problems and also for exhaustion and irritability as above from www.helios.com or good health shops.

MENOPAUSAL SYMPTOMS

There is a lot that you can do, from eating soy nuts to taking herbal remedies, before you reach for the HRT. I have no first-hand experience yet, so go to www.naturalhealthpractice.com and read the excellent *New Natural Alternatives to HRT* by Marilyn Glenville.

PREMENSTRUAL PROBLEMS

I'm a big believer in magnetic therapy for this. I wore a Bioflow bracelet (see www.ecoflow.com) and noticed the difference within two months. You can also wear a Ladycare magnet clipped to your knickers (from Lloyds Pharmacies), and of course think about your sanitary protection. It's not scientifically proven but I am convinced, along with many of my website forum members, that wearing a Mooncup (see www.mooncup.com) helps to regulate your periods and greatly reduces pain, particularly if you've switched from regular tampons (the theory is that tampons cause dryness and cramping).

It's a good idea to increase your magnesium levels. Make sure you're having lots of essential fatty acids, from foods like oily fish, and nuts and seeds. Some women find great benefit from taking the herbs agnus castus and dong quai. Visit your local independent health shop or nutritionist and ask for advice.

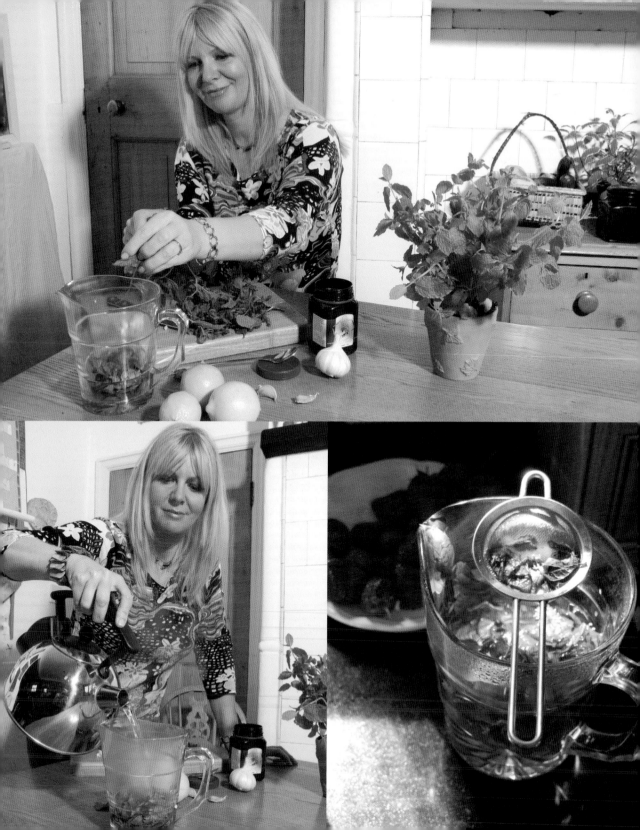

RASHES AND IRRITATED SKIN

See page 83 for more information on skincare, but for rashes and itchy skin conditions there's nothing finer than soothing porridge oats. Fill a little bag or thin sock with oats and run your bath water through it. The water will run 'milky' and you can use the oat filled bag as a 'flannel' all over the body. This is very soothing for children with chicken pox too.

SPLINTERS

If there's a problem with physical removal, put a tiny piece of good-quality bread on the splinter and tape it over with a plaster. The yeast in the bread is said to draw out the splinter.

STOMACH UPSETS

For poorly tums or nausea, fresh ginger is excellent; for debilitating morning sickness or travel sickness, nibble fresh ginger or even a ginger biscuit if you're on the go. You can buy ginger capsules in health shops too, and for children who suffer from travel sickness try the wrist bands that sit on the acupressure points, available from pharmacies.

For diarrhoea, sip water and if you can eat, eat some grated apple.

TOOTHACHE

You remember Oil of Cloves? Very old-style but well worth keeping in your natural medicine cabinet until you can get to see a dentist. For teething babies, crush a couple of homeopathic chamomilla tablets from Boots or **www.helios.com** on a spoon and rub it along the gums.

WARTS AND VERRUCAS

Tricky one this, as they will eventually go away on their own, but they can cause discomfort in the meantime. Homeopathy has good success with these problems; in general the remedy Thuja is good for warts.

For verrucas it sounds daft, but also try putting the inner side of a banana skin against the foot and taping it down with a plaster. Applying neat tea tree oil works well too.

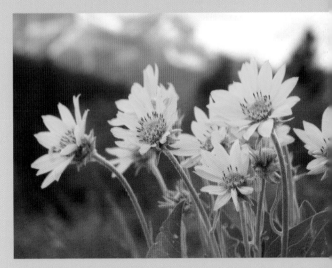

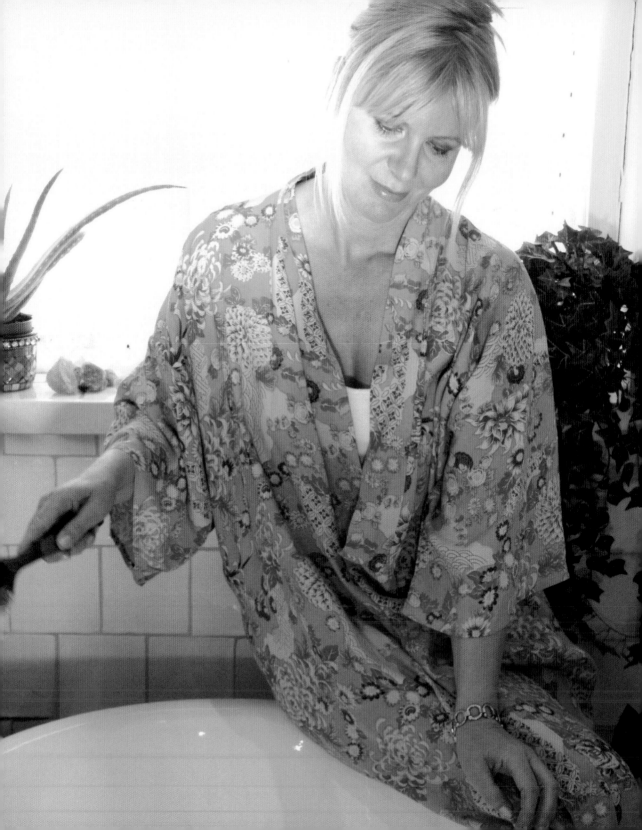

8 Personal Care

I appreciate you're probably asking, 'What difference does what I use on my face or hair make to the health and eco credentials of my home?' Well, more than you may think. There is information galore on chemical-free personal care in my book *Imperfectly Natural Woman* but there are a few basics I'd like to share with you here.

Just as the cupboard under the kitchen sink requires a lock when children are around, and most products display clearly their toxic dangers, so too should the average bathroom cabinet and the majority of the items inside it. The good news, though, is that there is now a natural alternative to just about everything.

For starters I'd say reduce the amount of personal care products you use anyway. Often we simply don't need four different preparations for our hair and three different types of moisturiser, one for cellulite, one for the décolletage (OK, I admit I've only just recently realised that's the bit above your boobs), a night cream for the neck . . . Virgin coconut oil does the lot for a fraction of the cost – more on this on page 87. Then set about reducing the number of man-made chemicals within the products you do use.

It's well documented that these can contribute to respiratory problems, poor concentration and falling sperm counts, and even in some cases can be carcinogenic. No one bottle of shampoo or moisturising lotion is going to make you ill, but I believe that the cumulative effect of hundreds of different chemicals almost certainly will, and the chemicals are damaging for the environment too.

So ditch your regular chemical-laden brands and replace with Fairtrade natural alternatives. Be careful of the word 'organic' on cosmetics and skincare – anyone can label their product organic or even use it in their brand name, even if the product contains perhaps only a tiny percentage of organic ingredients. My Romanian au pair proudly gave me a present – a bottle of shampoo that had written across it 'organic aloe vera natural shampoo'. I thanked her but then read the ingredients list, and yes, it contained about three per cent organic aloe vera and essential oil, but the rest was made up of a cocktail of potentially toxic synthetics.

If you want organic, make sure it's certified organic, preferably with the BDIH (Association of German Industries and Trading Firms for pharmaceuticals, health care products, food

'You can take no credit for beauty at sixteen. But if you are beautiful at sixty, it will be your soul's own doing.' Marie Carmichael Stopes, eugenist

supplements and personal hygiene products) or Soil Association logo.

There are now an increasing number of companies who have product ranges that are 100 per cent organic such as Spiezia Organics (www.spieziaorganics.com), Balm Balm (www.balmbalm.co.uk) and Essential Care (www.essential-care.co.uk). On my website directory (www.imperfectlynatural.com) I recommend many more great skincare companies whose products are 100 per cent natural, not tested on animals and many of them organic.

INGREDIENTS TO AVOID...

Parabens

These preservatives, found in many skincare and cosmetic products, are thought to be highly toxic and can cause hormone disruption and allergic reactions.

Sodium laurel sulphate

A foaming agent and harsh detergent found in toothpastes, shampoos and bubble baths, as well as in many cleaning products. It's a skin irritant and can be absorbed and cause damage to the eyes, brain, heart and liver.

Parfum

This is found in many guises in soaps, baby products and chemical cleaners. It can cause headaches, skin irritation and allergies. Artificial musks are also found in some baby wipes and air fresheners.

Pthalates

These pollutants can leak from products and be absorbed into our bodies. They are the hardest to avoid, as they're contained in so many products, from toys, even clothing made from PVC, through to furnishings, perfumes and cosmetics. They've been linked to a wide range of issues including fertility problems and altered hormone levels.

Alcohol and isopropyl

Found in hand lotions and after-shave fragrances, these are linked to depression, headaches and nausea.

Petrolatum or petro-based products

Often used in lip salves and baby oils, these are intended to rehydrate but can actually cause dryness and irritation.

I won't go on. I want to give you the positive approach!

MAKING THE SWITCH TO NATURAL PRODUCTS

Here are a few basic things to help you make the switch. It goes without saying that what you put on your skin not only affects you personally but will in due course be washed away into the

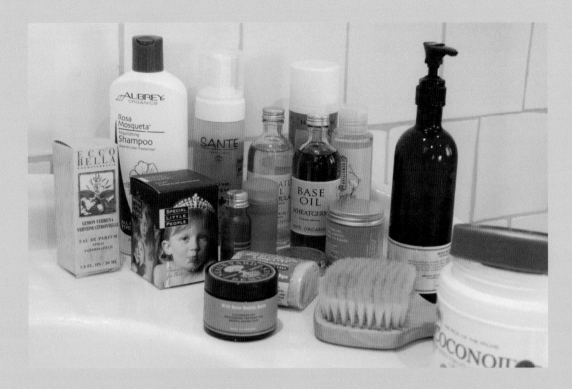

rivers and seas. I recommend some products to switch to, and if you're on a budget or feeling creative for most there's a simple version you can make at home. In some cases I've given you websites where you can locate these items, but many are readily available in good health stores.

SOAPS AND HAND WASHES

Castile soaps, made from vegetable oil – yes, the old-style ones – are great, as are natural soaps made with beeswax and using essential oils from fragrance. You can now buy beautiful natural soaps that make great gifts too.

I recommend:

Ethically traded and chemical-free soaps from **www.simplysoaps.com** and from **www.essentialspirit.co.uk**.

Dr Bronner's Castile soaps in health shops or from **www.kinetic4health.co.uk**.

Trevarno in Cornwall do lovely soaps **www.trevarno.co.uk**.

If you need something stronger, use the excellent Antibacterial Liquid Soap from Greenpeople (**www.greenpeople.co.uk**). Neem soap from **www.junglesale.com**.

Make your own

You can make your own liquid soaps easily by buying a bar of simple olive oil soap, such as Oliva from Holland and Barratt stores: grate it, and add boiling water and a couple of drops of essential oil if you like a fragrance – that's it. Pour it into a pump dispenser (you can buy one for as little as 40 pence) and you have easy-to-use, 100 per cent natural liquid soap that cost next to nothing. If it seems too gloopy, just add a bit more water.

BATHTIME

For the bath, avoid bubble baths – the chemicals used in most regular ones can be very drying – and soak a little muslin bag or sock filled with porridge oats in the water to soothe any irritated skin.   It feels as if you're bathing in milk, Cleopatra-style.

For everything natural and bathtime related, including towels, natural loofahs, Epsom salts and pumice stones, go to Eco Bath (**www.ecobath.co.uk**). There are excellent organic towels and linens form **www.greenfibres.com**. For a 'spa treatment' at home try w**ww.naturalspacompany.co.uk**.

TOOTHPASTES

The great fluoride debate is yet another whole book, I'm afraid, and not one I'll go into here, save to say I'm against fluoride (amongst other chemicals) in toothpaste, so look for fluoride-free natural toothpastes. You can get vegetarian non-fluoridated Ayurvedic tooth powders made from barks, herbs and flowers, but the best over-the-counter options, available in most health shops and some chemists, are:

Green People – particularly their children's Mandarin toothpaste – is excellent (**www.greenpeople.co.uk**) and kingfisher and Jason toothpaste from **www.kinetic4 health.co.uk**. The Miessence cosmetic range has a great natural lemon one, available by mail order from **www.sheerorganics.com**.

Of course for travelling when there's no water or toothpaste available get a natural toothbrush, only a couple of quid, and it will last for ages. It's basically a 'twig' from the root of the arrak tree and contains natural minerals. When you trim or peel back the bark it reveals a little natural brush and it's excellent for massaging the gums. Read about them at **www.naturaltoothbrush.com** and **www.thegreenstoreonline.co.uk**.

Make your own
....

Make your own toothpaste by mixing a paste of bicarb, salt, a little water and lemon juice. Tastes slightly odd, but very cheap and with zero nasties, and you get used to it.

BODY MOISTURISERS

If you haven't read my other books or heard me speak at events, you may not know of this absolute gem of a tip. It's a health-giving, money-saving, fairly traded natural wonder: coconut oil.

They do say don't put anything on your skin that you can't eat, and though I'm imperfect in many areas, here's one where I practise what I preach. I don't tend to use it on my face, but it's fantastic for almost all skin types as an all-over body moisturiser, and it's not greasy. Actually it doesn't really smell of coconuts. It's a wonderful hair conditioner too.

It's also a functional food and one of the healthiest oils to use in cooking, although it does give a richer taste, so I just use less. You can buy it very cheaply as cooking oil in food stores that stock Asian and Caribbean foods, and from **www.revital.co.uk,** for as little as £2.00. My favourite is a little more expensive, but it's virgin coconut oil fairly traded from Sri Lanka, and some of the profits are put back into local sustainable projects. See **www.coconoil.com.**

If you like a fragrance, you can still use coconut oil. For a heavenly fragrance, go to **www.sensitiveskincareco.com** for their Gardenia Scented Coconut Oil.

For other natural body moisturisers I particularly like, see:

www.akamuti.co.uk

www.naturalskincarecompany.com

– I like their Paul Penders intensive care therapy.

www.absolutelypure.co.uk

www.rawgaia.com

For the décolletage, the gel from Neal's Yard Remedies (**www.nealsyardremedies.com**) is fantastic.

MSM lotion is also hugely underrated. Methylsulfonylmethane is the base and there are usually other natural ingredients added to make a really rich lotion which helps elasticity and is anti-ageing; it is available from **www.highernature.co.uk.**

FOR YOUR FACE

'Nothing prevents one from appearing natural as the desire to appear natural.'

François de La Rochefoucauld, author

Coconut oil may be heavy for most complexions, but I still believe that facial oils are the way to go for most people. I've tried many expensive creams and night creams over the years, all proudly shouting their anti-ageing properties and their vitamin fixes, but one by one most of them have brought me out in zits. Facial oils are therapeutic on many levels and if you can find a good aromatherapist, ask them to make up a blend especially for you. There are lots of excellent ones on the market too, including the one from Green People (**www.greenpeople.co.uk**) and the gorgeous organic orange flower facial oil from **www.nealsyardremedies.com.**

Balms are also lovely and some people find them easier to use than oils. Try **www.spieziaorganics.com** or Burts Bees, available in good pharmacies.

If it's just got to be a cream or lotion, there are some wonderful rich 100 per cent natural ones such as the gorgeous Hemega 3 range from **www.lemonburst.co.uk**. The gentle creams from **www.purenuffstuff.co.uk** and the Martina Gebhart Happy Ageing Cream from **www.trueaffinity.co.uk.**

Make your own

Again you can use simple olive oil or hemp oil

as an excellent facial moisturiser; just use it sparingly. You can make your own facial oil by using 30 ml of jojoba or cold pressed grape seed oil as a base in a glass bottle and, using a dropper, adding 5–15 drops of lavender, rose, myrrh, geranium, whatever takes your fancy. If you are suffering from a cold or respiratory problems, use eucalyptus. To buy the basics, and for info, go to **www.eoco.org.uk**.

Always check for contraindications when using essential oils, particularly if you're pregnant or breastfeeding.

When your skin is feeling very dry or seems dull or flaky, treat yourself to a face mask. I like the Organic White Tea Facemask from

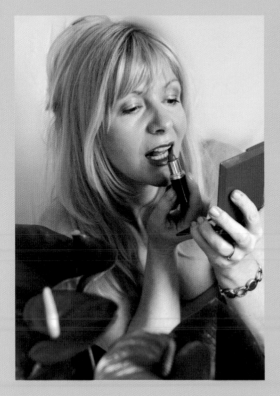

www.nealsyardremedies.com.

There's also the Home Facial from Paul Penders, and some wonderful natural facial treatments, from the Natural Skincare Company (**www.naturalskincarecompany.com**).

Make your own

It's easy to make your own exfoliator: just use oatmeal, rub it gently over your face and wash off. You can mix it with honey for a really good facial scrub. For a face pack, see what the fresh leftovers are in the fridge. Avocado, honey, any fresh soft fruits all make wonderful face packs. Egg white can be used if you want a 'stiffening' pack, and for a toner, swish rose water (available from chemists) over your face.

SUNSCREEN

Best of all, cover up! Regular sunscreen contains a horrifying cocktail of chemicals that some say are far worse than a dose of sunshine. Remember years ago heliotherapy was the order of the day? But of course I'm not recommending lying out in the hottest part of day, exposed to the harsh rays. Wear big hats and sunglasses, carry an old-style parasol and dress children in sun protective clothing.

For those occasions when you must use a sun cream, opt for a natural one. Zinc and titanium oxide sunscreens are the best. My favourite is from **www.urtekram.de**, and also I like Badger sun block (**www.badgerbalm .co.uk**); both are available in some health shops. For great sun creams for babies and children go to **www.greenpeople.co.uk**.

Make your own

To make your own – well, you can buy simple zinc cream. You'll have surfer-style white nose, but that's okay!

For mild sunburn, use neat lavender oil. If you just think you've had a tad too much sun, try Green People's After Sun moisturising cream.

SHAMPOOS AND CONDITIONERS

The list of recommended companies is growing daily but one of the few certified organic ones is by Essential Care (**www.essential-care.co.uk**). Other personal favourites include Aubrey Organics' Rose Mosqueta shampoo and conditioner (**www.aubreyorganics.co.uk**).

For hairspray, mousses and conditioning treatments, look at Sante products from **www.santecosmetics.co.uk** and Lavera from **www.lavera.co.uk**.

Make your own

You can make simple excellent home-made conditioner and treatments. A few drops of essential oil of rosemary mixed with a teaspoon of sweet almond oil is excellent for psoriasis and dandruff. Gently massage and leave for half an hour before rinsing out. Avocado with a little coconut milk makes a great conditioner.

Chamomile flowers mixed with lemon juice is great for lifting blonde hair. Steep the flowers in warm water, mix in the lemon juice, and use as a rinse. Do that regularly and you'll really notice a difference after a couple of weeks.

You can buy chamomile flowers from the Journal of Chinese Medicine (**www.jcm.co.uk**).

DEODORANTS

Deodorants have hit the headlines, and this is a subject I've been talking about for years. Regular deodorants and antiperspirants have been proved to be detrimental to the environment and, worryingly, research also shows that in breast cancer patients high levels of aluminium residue were found in the breast tissue. Now scientists may argue that much of the absorbed aluminium is from our food stuffs, but I would argue that in fact it comes from deodorants. It's of particular concern for women around the under arm area, where the sensitive lymph nodes need to be allowed to drain, not to be blocked. It's known to cause cancer in animal models but in my view aluminium is not the only issue with regular deodorants. It's important that we remember what else is in most of them – just about everything in that 'scary chemicals to avoid' list! It's actually a very bad idea to try to stop the body perspiring as we need to perspire in order to expel toxins and regulate our body temperature. Interestingly it's not the sweat that smells; only when bacteria forms do we get whiffy, so the way natural deodorants work is not to inhibit perspiration but to create an environment where bacteria can't thrive. Crystal deodorants work by leaving a fine layer of mineral salts on the skin, which is not greasy or sticky and has no fragrance. They're cheap, last for ages and are 100 per cent natural. They come in sprays or roll-ons and they work on zits too! Just wet the stone or stick slightly and apply to spot. I like those from **www.littlesatsuma.com**, and Pitrok, sold in many health stores and at **www.pitrok.co.uk**.

If you prefer a spray, or roll-on with a fragrance but still want to be natural, there are now some excellent natural deodorants such as the lemon and coriander one from **www.nealsyardremedies.com**.

Then there's the Amazing Body Stick from **www.naturalcollection.com**. Don't ask me how this seemingly inert stick of stainless steel neutralises odours, but it works! It costs £20 but lasts a lifetime.

Make your own

Control your body odour by drinking lots of water and consider limiting processed foods, spices, alcohol and sugar. What you eat greatly affects your perspiration. Bathe and shower without using synthetic chemicals, and a quick wipe around with a fresh lemon works too (make sure you don't put it back for the salad dressing, though!).

You can also make your own with half a cup of jojoba oil and a few drops of bergamot essential oil and one drop of tea tree oil. Store it in a pump dispenser.

FOR THE GUYS

Pretty much everything mentioned above is suitable for guys too. The male grooming market has increased massively, so men, do think about your chemical usage. It's not enough just to slap on any old shaving cream, followed by a chemical aftershave, and then spray on an antiperspirant before heading off to be an eco warrior.

Several companies now offer a natural men's range. If you want sleek packaging and great aftershave stuff and moisturising lotions, look at Flintedge (**www.flintedge.com**).

An excellent men's range is available also from **www.nealsyardremedies.com** (who also offer men's holistic facials in some of their UK branches); **www.livingnature.com** do an excellent shower wash and **www.greenpeople.co.uk** have a full men's grooming range.

Watch this space for *Imperfectly Natural Man* . . .

MAKE-UP AND COSMETICS

Of course, in an ideal world we wouldn't need to wear any! There some excellent ranges now from:

www.lavera.co.uk
www.livingnature.co.uk.

Gorgeous bright-coloured mineral eye shadows from **www.lilylolo.co.uk**. Great lipsticks in cute cases with a mirror from **www.lemonburst.co.uk**.

I've also just found a great range of mineral

cosmetics that are certified 100 per cent vegan and cruelty-free: www.inikacosmetics.com.

FRAGRANCES

Once you stop using chemicals you may find you don't feel the need to wear perfumes any more, but for a treat try the natural lemon one from www.lemonburst.co.uk. There's also a range of natural perfumes at www.florame. co.uk.

One favourite is the Pur Arome Eau de Parfum made using only natural and nature-identical ingredients from the excellent Anne Maria Borlind www.annemarieborlind.co.uk. If you're lucky enough to be visiting India, try and source an ayervedic medicine that's also a 100 per cent perfume in powder form.

You can get lovely 'pick me up' roll-on sticks, perfect for travelling and containing essential oils. I love the peppermint one from www.akamuti.co.uk.

Make your own

That's easy – dab a tiny drop of essential oil on your wrist. Patchouli is kind of sensual and 'hippy-ish'. If you can afford it, rose is very feminine and classy.

NAIL POLISH

Most regular nail polishes contain a scary mix of touluene, formaldehyde and solvents – not advised! Fortunately there are now full-colour ranges of water-based polishes and acetone-free polish removers available from www.suvarna.co.uk.

If you're lucky enough to be near Herefordshire, check out www.greenhands.co.uk for a totally green and natural manicure using natural products.

SANITARY PROTECTION

The average home absolutely does not need tampons flushed down the loos or indeed put into the waste-bin to add to landfill.

Some regular sanitary protection is bleached and contains potentially carcinogenic chemicals. If you want to use tampons, opt for the organic ones from www.natracare.co.uk. They make towels and maternity pads too. Even better, use organic washable menstrual pads from www.drapersorganiccotton.co.uk.

Best and cheapest of all, use a Mooncup (www.mooncup.co.uk).

'There is no cosmetic for beauty like happiness.'
Marguerite Blessington, countess, author

9 Children

'Behold the child, by nature's kindly law, pleased with a rattle, tickled with a straw.' Alexander Pope, poet

It is interesting that so many of us only begin to take a personal interest in being a bit more natural and green when we become parents for the first time. Certainly I was concerned about eating healthily, considering supplements and even recognising the impact of my spirituality and my thoughts on my health and well-being; but it wasn't until I had my first child that I started to realise I may wish to leave some of the planet behind for future generations, to which I was now contributing – and yes, it absolutely was my responsibility.

Even then I must confess I came to it from a selfish standpoint. I was considering whether to use re-usable nappies, and rather than simply being swayed by the frightening statistics of eight million nappies per day in landfill taking over 200 years to biodegrade (which, let's face it, ought to have been enough to help me make my choice), my real concern was for my babies' skin and the potential toxicity of the super-absorbent gel within the disposable nappies. The good news is that even for selfish imperfect types like me, there is often an environmental benefit associated with just about every 'natural health' choice you make.

I would say limit your purchases. It is so easy to get carried away and buy every last bit of baby equipment that the advertisers would have you believe is essential. Stop and think before buying the latest must-have buggy or pram. Check local 'nearly new' shops and parenting forums, where you'll often find your favourite model at a fraction of the price. Remember, too, that babies are happier and sleep longer, and you are 'hands-free', if you carry them in a baby carrier (sling).

If you haven't considered it before, now is really the time to switch your laundry products. That precious baby skin just can't be red and irritated by harsh detergents, so switch to gentle eco brands or, better still, soapnuts (see page 24).

Never spray chemical sprays anywhere near babies or children, and make sure you clean areas where they're crawling or eating with chemical-free cleaning products. 'How?' I hear you say. 'I need something antibacterial, surely?' Well, for certain things, of course, but make it naturally antibacterial. Use an e-cloth (see page 15) and a drop of tea tree oil, and to clean the surfaces of high chairs, use the wonderful totally natural All-Purpose Nursery Cleaner from **www.babyscents.co.uk** or the organic chemical-free Surface Spa from **www.natural-house.co.uk** (see also page 15).

Babycare really is another whole book, and all my views on breastfeeding, nappies, first foods, and all things baby and young children-esque are

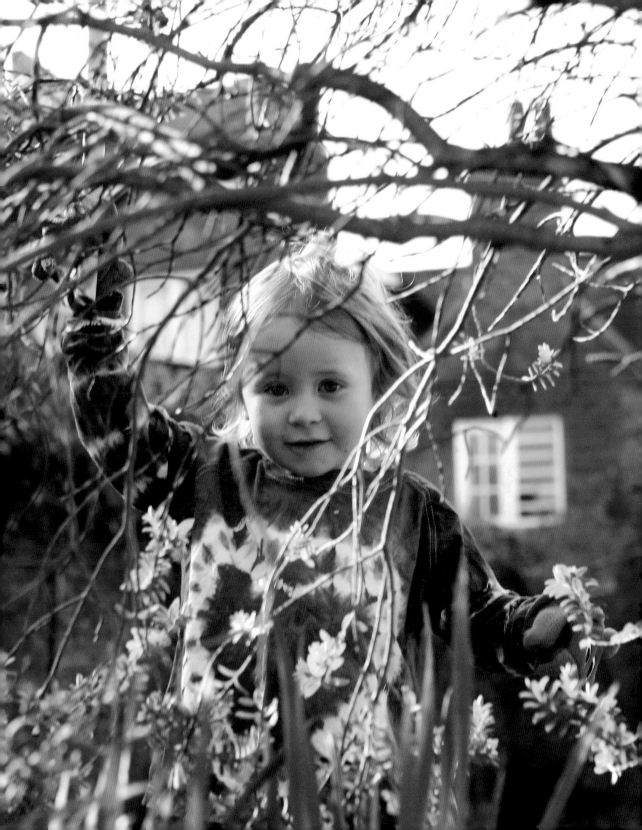

well documented in *Imperfectly Natural Baby and Toddler.*

BABY SKINCARE

Remember you don't need to use much more than plain water for the first month, and even after that you can top and tail a baby but they don't need to bathe every day. The chlorine in the water can be too drying for a baby's sensitive skin. Consider a dechlorination ball for the bath from www.sensitiveskincareco.com.

You definitely don't need harsh soaps for a baby's skin. Use baby products from one of the natural companies, such as the Organic Babies range from www.greenpeople.co.uk, the lovely range that includes the aptly named Bum Spray from www.greenface.co.uk or the nappy rash creams from www.purepotions.co.uk. Other excellent websites offering natural baby products include www.cecebaby.co.uk and www.delicateskin.co.uk.

HAIR-WASHING

Some babies and young children hate having their hair washed. With my first child I feared the whole street could hear the screams when I attempted it. By my second child I'd realised his hair didn't actually need washing – there's another whole book to write on how wonderful hair is when not washed, but that may be a bridge too far. As a rule, however, babies and young children need to wash their hair very infrequently. When you do want to, it's against

my better nature to recommend a 'gimmick' but the shampoo Rinse Aid 'jug' from www.trendykid.co.uk is fantastic and really does keep water out of their eyes.

NAPPIES

Go washable: it's easier than you think. Or if you're in imperfect mode on this one, there are some great eco brands such as Moltex Oko and Tushies. Natracare make excellent baby wipes.

For advice on a full range of nappies and accessories, see www.thenappylady.com.

CLOTHES

Kids grow out of their clothes so quickly that buying second-hand can be a very sensible option. I kitted mine out for years with second-hand clothes.

If you're going to buy new, opt for organic cotton or natural fabrics. You'll find the quality much better and you'll be able to use them for younger siblings or indeed pass them on or lend to your friends.

Frugi (www.welovefrugi.com) makes a fantastic range for babies and children with a generous cut for babies in cloth nappies.

Other great companies who make eco clothes for kids include Tatty Bumpkin (www.tattybumpkin.co.uk) and Stella James (www.stella-james.co.uk).

You can buy fabulous soft leather first shoes from www.starchildshoes.co.uk.

SCHOOL UNIFORMS

Buying new school clothes is astronomically expensive and fortunately the tide is turning. There is no longer any stigma attached to buying second-hand; in fact it's recognised as being a sensible, sustainable choice. Uniform2 (**www.uniform2.com**) offer a great nationwide resource for good condition second-hand uniforms.

TOYS

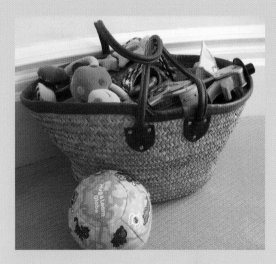

Ditch the expensive excessively packaged bright plastic toys and let this be one area where you really save money and tick the reduce, reuse and recycle box. Good-quality, second-hand toys are available in abundance. Just make sure they're clean and safe (a great tip for 'sterilising' soft toys is to put them inside a plastic bag and leave them in the freezer for a few hours). You'll notice that babies and young children really don't mind that they aren't shiny and new.

See if you have a local toy library. You can usually borrow items for a couple of pounds and keep them for a few weeks, and often after three weeks of whizzing round on that bright plastic toy car, many a toddler will realise he didn't need to own it after all. If you have an older child wanting a bike or another expensive item, then scour car boot sales and look on Freecycle (see page 15). I've found a child's motorbike and all manner of great toys for a fraction of their new cost that way.

If you want to buy new, opt for environmentally friendly toys made from organic cotton and natural fabrics for soft toys (such as the gorgeous fluffy organic ones from **www.ecochums.com**).

Look for wooden toys made from wood from sustainably managed forests, which is really hard-wearing. If you do buy plastic, be particularly wary of PVC toys because babies will chew whatever fits in their mouth, and be careful of potentially toxic paint too. There have been toys made by well-known brands recalled because of dangerous levels of lead in their paint. Opt for toys with plant-based dyes or paints such as those from ethical companies: see **www.ninnynoodlenoo.com** or **www.holtztoys.co.uk**.

For all manner of sustainable toys and art and craft materials, go to **www.myriadonline.co.uk**. They offer plant-based paints containing no toxic chemicals, beautiful block beeswax crayons which last for ages (and don't contain petroleum as the regular ones do), as well as 'fairy' wool and art materials in vibrant colours.

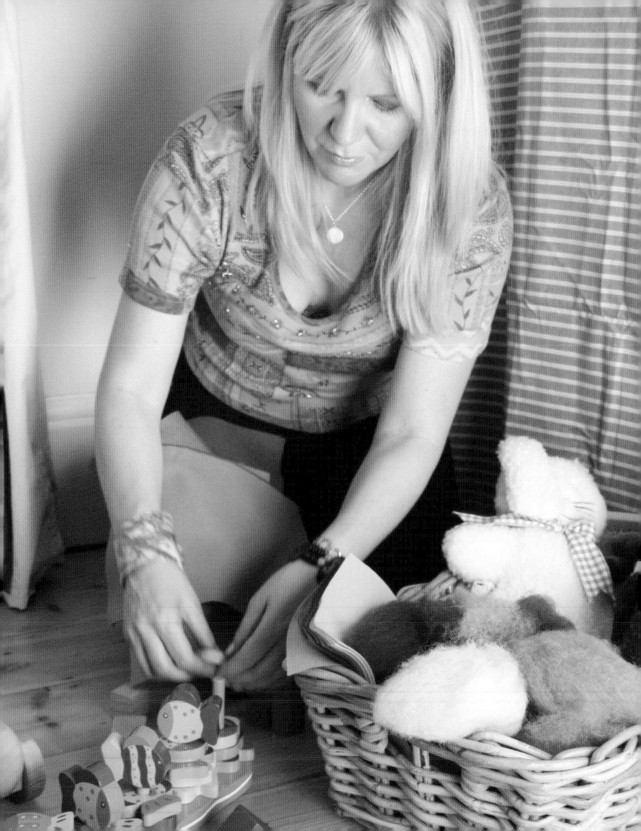

SIMPLE CRAFTS AND ACTIVITIES

Think back to when you were young. I'll bet you made a tambourine from bottle tops and a shaker from a yoghurt pot containing dried peas. Simple activities that cost next to nothing are the new Barbie dolls. Kids love fashioning something new from something old. Inspire them by showing them some of the wonderful recycled items around now, such as the great range of office stationery with a notebook that says 'I used to be a juice carton' and a mouse mat that declares proudly, 'I used to be a car tyre.' Of course, kids don't have the resources to melt down plastic chips and process into line fibre, but they can be extremely creative by turning an old car tyre into a planter or decorating a picture frame from a collection of bottle tops. Make a doll's house from a big cardboard box, keep some old hats and clothes for a dressing-up box – the possibilities are endless.

Buy natural water paint in just three colours – red, blue and yellow. From these primary colours there's a wonderful art lesson to be had from mixing all the other shades the children need.

Baking and cooking with kids is great fun. Look for child-sized chopping boards and round-edged knives, and get the children involved in planning a meal, cooking it and preparing the table, adding a few flowers from the garden in a jar. Growing their own organic veg will almost certainly result in them wanting to eat it. For the impatient, see page 33 [gardening section] and **www.rocketgardens.co.uk**; and growing herbs and sprouts (see page 37) is simple and very rewarding.

Of course, best of all is to be outside with children of all ages. Get used to putting wellies on and pottering about in parks, woods, rivers and streams in all weathers. Even a busy street on a rainy day can prove delightful with a young child – just join in with them and jump in all the puddles.

You can make all manner of toys and activities from tree stumps, logs and branches and help children appreciate the seasons by making paper kites and May baskets (paper cones filled with wild flowers) in spring, making a chain from daisies and berry picking in the summer, weaving wheat straw decorations and carving pumpkins in the autumn, and making pine cone bird feeders and firelighters in the winter.

If this is an area that interests you, go to **www.brighterblessings.co.uk** for a wealth of ideas for crafts, and I highly recommend the book *Earthwise Environmental: Crafts and Activities with Young Children* by Carol Petrash.

'Parents are often so busy with the physical rearing of children that they miss the glory of parenthood, just as the grandeur of the trees is lost when raking leaves.' Marcelene Cox, writer

Imperfectly natural home Q&A

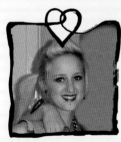

Holly Lloyd
Fashion student (Bristol)

Describe your home. Mid-terraced Victorian house, small patio garden, four bedrooms, a lounge, a bathroom and a toilet, dining area/bike storage!

How would you describe your interior 'style' and furnishings? Mis-matched and studenty, cosy, feminine, friendly and YELLOW!

What does your home mean to you? As a student home I think it's important to make it feel as homely as possible. We have filled the place with quirky objects and possessions, pictures, plants, lights and general crap! But all these things make the difference between a dwelling and a home. We all try to act like a family to make living together fun and supportive. Our door is always open.

Have you attempted any eco DIY or modifications for a greener home? Nothing structural as it is a rented house, but we do make a conscious effort to live eco in other ways.

How would your home rate for energy-efficiency? What have you done to reduce energy usage? When you buy new appliances, do you consider the energy-efficiency? Fairly good, we don't buy our own appliances but are conscious about the ones we use, we wash on 30, share loads, don't use the heating unless it's absolutely necessary (put layers on instead), we don't use much water, we don't have a dishwasher or tumble dryer, we only boil the kettle with the amount of water we need.

How 'eco' are your furniture, floorings and furnishings? Not very, although nothing's been changed in years so at least nothing's gone to the tip!

What cleaning/laundry/stain removing products do you use? Ecover washing powder and surface spray, all other products are standard supermarket brands.

If you could buy any one 'eco' gadget or item for your home inside or out what would it be? Solar panels.

What kind of cookware do you use? Whatever ends up in our cupboards!

What's your best tip for getting your fridge and larder stocked with good healthy food? We try to share our meals, we shop for our veg at a fruit and veg stall down the road that sells local produce, most other food comes from Aldi but there is a lovely organic and health food shop too, which we treat ourselves to when we can afford it! We walk to all of these shops.

What about composting? Bristol is brilliant about recycling and all our food waste gets collected from our door.

What do you regularly recycle? How? Our recycling gets collected weekly, they take paper and card, glass, cans and food waste (unfortunately not plastics).

If you have a garden what are your eco tips? After trimming the hedges, put the clippings back on the garden to decompose.

What are your views on the possible dangers of electro 'smog'/wifi/emfs etc.? Have you taken any protective measures for you and your family? Don't know enough about this subject and have done nothing about it.

Do you know your carbon footprint and do you care about it? (Be honest!) I care very much and try to be conscious of it when I go about doing things in everyday life.

How green are you – lime/olive? Rotten cabbage green!

Do you have an imperfectly natural guilty secret? Many! I feel guilty about toiletry products: don't use 'eco-friendly' brands or feel drawn to them.

What would your dream home be like?
A place where everyone feels welcome.

What are your top three tips for a naturally healthy home?
Recycle EVERYTHING you possibly can.
Shop local, local produce.
Cook from scratch … no ready meals.

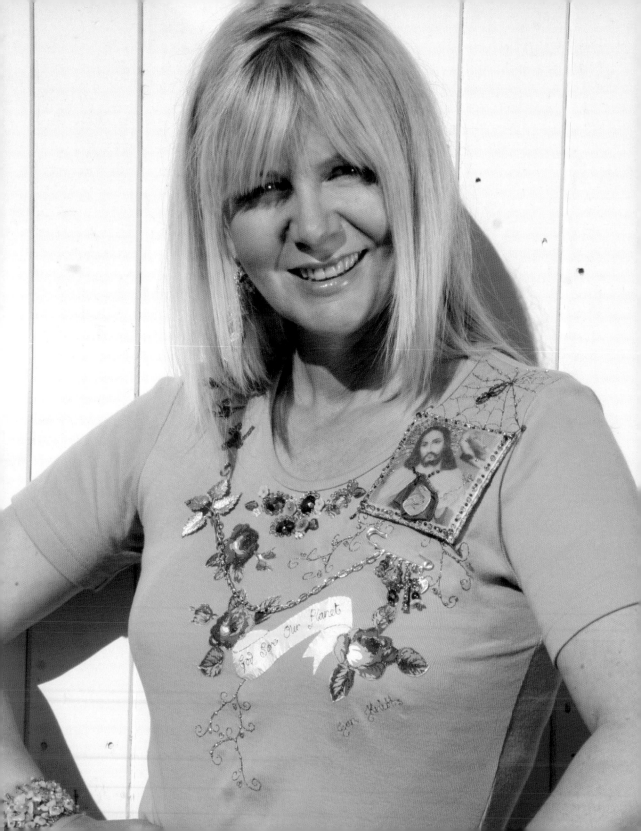

10 Clothing, furnishings and fabrics

CLOTHES

We all know it's a good idea to wash your clothes less, reduce the temperature of the wash, use eco detergents, avoid tumble dryers and too much ironing (that one's never been an issue for me) and if an item must be dry cleaned opt for Green Earth or similar (see page 29). But what about the actual clothes themselves? Don't panic. I'm not about to try to tell you what styles and colours you should be wearing this season – though I do believe wearing certain colours absolutely affects your mood (and in this respect, the ubiquitous black is not a good colour to wear). However, I am going to try to persuade you to think about your 'footprint' and your ethics when buying your wardrobe.

There are various factors to take into account when it comes to whether or not our clothing is 'ethical'. We're all aware of the controversy surrounding real fur, but what about the humble T-shirt? It never ceases to amaze me that we all check our food ingredients, and buy organic, yet when it comes to the average T-shirt we are totally unaware that it contains GM cotton, and has been treated with a staggering amount of pesticides and is most certainly not Fairtrade or sustainable.

People Tree (**www.peopletree.co.uk**), which is an ethical company that uses organic cotton, has researched this in great detail and its findings show that only 2.5 per cent of all farmland worldwide is under cotton, but a staggering 10 per cent of chemical pesticides and 22 per cent of all insecticides sprayed are on cotton. Most cotton is heavily irrigated. The Aral Sea has almost disappeared as the watercourses that flowed into it have been diverted to grow –'white gold' –in Uzbekistan and Kazakhstan. This has been catastrophic for the fishery and is now destroying the cotton fields, as years of rapid evaporation from semi-desert soils has left salt residues, making the land unfertile.

On top of this, when you learn about the conditions people work in the production of

'The origins of clothing are not practical. They are mystical and erotic. The primitive man in the wolf-pelt was not keeping dry; he was saying: Look what I killed. Aren't I the best?' Katharine Hamnett

cotton, the toxic chemicals they are exposed to, the wages they are paid and their lack of prospects, you realise that low-cost clothing actually comes with a very high price indeed.

There are now ethical trade initiatives. For instance, Labour Behind the Label (www.labourbehindthelabel.org) traces the whole process and ensures that that organic T-shirt really is 100 per cent fairly traded from start to finish.

The great news is that there's so much more available that is 'ethical' and yet still looks good. A few years back when I wrote my first book, it was a different story: there were only a handful of designers who were producing ethical clothes and in truth they were usually

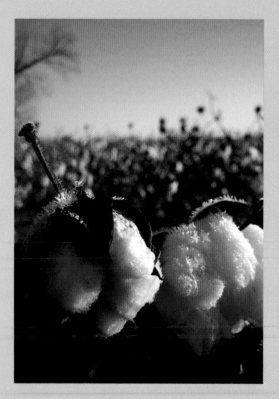

fairly bland. Now there are a whole host of bright and funky items using more sustainable natural organic textiles such as hemp, bamboo and 100 per cent organic cotton, some of it in high street chains like M&S and Top Shop.

It's not just the source of the fabric that needs to be considered for its environmental impact: if the dyes used on the textiles are chemical-based then you can be almost back at square one.

In *The New Green Consumer Guide* by Julia Hayles, the author states this fascinating fact: 'In the Middle Ages, hatters (people who made and dyed hats) often used some pretty nasty substances in their colour-fixing dyes. They didn't wear protective clothing and some of them absorbed so many toxic chemicals and heavy metals that they became deranged. That's where the expression "mad as a hatter" comes from.'

Look for plant-based dyes wherever possible and consider the way you shop for clothes.

If you want to buy new, look at labels such as:

People Tree (www.peopletree.co.uk)

Eco Eco (www.eco-eco.co.uk)

Piccalilly www.piccalilly.co.uk

Gossypium www.gossypium.co.uk

If you want to splash out on high fashion eco style, look at;

www.katharinehamnett.com

Eco couture from www.fashionpublic.com

Eco – Colin Firth's London shop www.eco-age.com

If you want something really special, find someone who will create something bespoke using recycled and ethical materials. See the picture on page 100, where I'm wearing a really funky embroidered T-shirt and earrings made by the very talented Jan Knibbs (www.janknibbs.com) from recycled materials. Her company is called 'Something Old, Something New'. They'll make you anything from a T-shirt to a wedding dress made from recycled materials with hand-embroidered embellishments.

For babies and children there's a wealth of choice of organic and Fairtrade clothing. To name just a few:

www.welovefrugi.com
www.stella-james.co.uk
www.tattybumpkin.co.uk

Jeans

For jeans, look at www.sharkachakra.com. The company uses organic denim, dyed naturally and fairly traded. Not cheap, though, at £200. I prefer to scour charity shops for really old jeans that are still wearing well.

Bags and shoes

For shoes, look at ethical companies such as Beyond Skin (www.beyondskin.co.uk) and the lovely ethical handmade shoes available from www.greenshoes.co.uk.

For re-usable bags, see page 51.

For handbags and backpacks, you can now be chic and still eco with a bag made from recycled bottles or car tyres – see the ranges from www.naturalcollection.com.

You can of course buy vintage shoes and bags from vintage stores and auction sites, prolonging their life even further.

CLOTHES SWAP

If you fancy a change of wardrobe, organise a clothes swap party with your friends. Often that pinstripe dress you paid a fortune for but never wore will be perfect for the new neighbour at No. 23, and perhaps that red linen dress of your cousin's which you've always coveted could be yours if she's worn it just too many times in public.

MAKE DO AND MEND

It seems very old-style to think of repairing an item these days, but often we can elongate the life of good clothing by a few stitches or adding some different buttons. There are fantastic suggestions in *Make Do and Mend: Keeping Family and Home Afloat on War Rations*. For more up-to-date tips, go to www.sewing.about.com, and you'll find some great ideas too on www.craftster.org.

'Beware of all enterprises that require new clothes.'

Henry David Thoreau, philosopher

FURNISHINGS

Stylish yet eco and affordable furniture and home furnishings are more difficult to source than fashionable eco clothing. Years ago our parents probably saved up for a decent three-piece suite and a few items of wooden furniture and that was usually it until at least their 50th wedding anniversary. Today, home furnishings have become much more disposable and sometimes we don't stop to think if something can be repaired or adapted rather than discarded.

CURTAINS

Curtains are certainly an area of debate because they do need to be good quality, heavy and well lined for good insulation, but the production of such items is extremely expensive in terms of labour and energy costs. If possible, opt for second-hand ones. Go to www.thecurtainexchange.net, which has high-quality curtains at bargain prices. Having said that, in rooms where insulation is not an issue, forget heavy curtains altogether and opt for strips of simple muslin or thin organic cotton. They can just be tied to a curtain pole, which gives a lovely dreamy effect.

Remember, when it comes to home furnishings it's often a balance between thrift and beauty. But if you want something new but truly eco opt for hemp. Draper's Organic (www.drapersorganic.co.uk) do excellent hemp curtains and also hemp shower curtains (hemp is perfect in that situation as it doesn't allow any mould).

FURNITURE

If you're buying wooden furniture or indeed any wood in the hardware store, always look for the FSC stamp (the Forest Stewardship Council is an international organisation dedicated to promoting responsible management of forests). It's also a good idea, particularly if an item does not feature the FSC symbol, to check the conservation status of the wood you're buying to check if it's endangered or vulnerable. Friends of the Earth have a 'good wood' guide on their website (www.foe.org).

In the south-east, buy locally grown timber from www.woodnet.org.uk.

For more on wood and natural floorings, see page 126.

You could opt for something very original such as furniture made from recycled glass. Greenapple have a fantastic range of tables and storage units, available at www.furnituretoday.co.uk, and will even take commissions.

'Perhaps believing in good design is like believing in God, it makes you an optimist.' Sir Terence Conran

FABRICS IN THE HOME

An unholy amount of toxic chemicals are used in the preparation of flame retardants, which by law had to be applied to all new textiles, including mattresses, foam beds, curtains, blinds and loose and fitted sofa and chair covers manufactured after 1988. Perhaps the impact of some house fires has been reduced, but the impact on our health and the environment is significant. Brominated flame retardants are chemicals with a long life span, remaining in our bodies and potentially causing hormone disruption. If you buy new, check the manufacturer's policy about flame retardant chemicals. It's not compulsory for the labels on textiles to indicate that the fabrics have been treated with formaldehyde resins and other chemicals. If you're unsure, allow furniture covers or mattress to 'off-gas' for a while in a well-ventilated room before use if possible.

If you're buying new, look for upholstery made from natural fibres such as linen, wool, hemp and cotton. Also be aware of the foam fillings in chair and scatter cushions: synthetic fillings such as polyurethane foam are manufactured using chemicals such as isocyanates and diisocynates (NCO), which can cause asthma and other respiratory issues. Many people are allergic to feather and down too; a better bet for fillings is unbleached cotton and wool, preferably organic and untreated. Remember that if you're getting chair cushions re-upholstered too. **www.bluebanyan.co.uk** sell a range of fillings, including buckwheat.

For duvets, one of my best buys recently was a 100 per cent silk-filled duvet, incredibly light yet warm. Perfect for anyone suffering from allergies. They do silk sheets, cot bedding and pillows too at amazing prices. **www.serenitysilk.co.uk**

Look for furnishings that carry the EU eco label – to qualify for this they have to contain no flame retardant chemicals that are harmful to the environment and health and be designed to be taken apart and be recycled.

There are other criteria that apply to all manufacturers who produce a wide range of items – look at **www.eco-label.com**.

If your upholstered furniture is worn, just replace the covers to bring the item up to date, or add some cushions with covers made from recycled fabrics to bring an individual touch. You can either buy second-hand fabric or adapt clothes or fabric you have lying around.

CLEANING FURNISHINGS

When sofas or chairs look a bit grubby, don't think of reaching for chemical cleaning solutions. For heavy curtains, sofas, carpets and even walls, you won't find anything more effective than a steam cleaner. Hire or borrow one and give them a good blast. For stains on fabric, try the Ecover stain remover, and for stains on the carpet try to remove as quickly as possible; soda water works as a good spot stain remover, as does bicarbonate of soda. For more on green cleaning, see page 12.

11 Organising and clutter-clearing

'Realise what you really want. It stops you from chasing butterflies and puts you to work digging gold.'

William Moulton Marsden, psychologist

FENG SHUI

After you've battled with trying to pronounce it, the next problem with feng shui is trying to work out what the hell it is and whether it really is relevant to us here in the West. The name translates as 'wind and water' and this ancient Chinese art has been used for over 3,000 years to determine the most auspicious sites to place important buildings and even whole cities.

In the UK we really only skim the surface of this incredibly complex art by using a kind of Westernised version of it in order to try to bring some 'luck' into our lives and to decide upon the best placement of furniture and furnishings.

All cosmic stuff aside, I believe feng shui is relevant to us, because an eco house is a healthy house, and in the same way that a home full of harmful synthetic chemicals can make you sick, so can a house full of 'stuck' or stale energy. All things have an energy, and our surroundings and possessions are important, not only acting as a barometer to our own personal issues but metaphorically exacerbating situations and feelings we may perhaps want to avoid. Feng shui attempts to expose the symbolism in everything we surround ourselves with, and show us practical ways of 'clearing the space', thereby enabling us to move forward to new opportunities in our lives.

Some may want to delve deeper into the ancient Chinese philosophies, but in my imperfect world, I have no problem with just taking the bits of feng shui I find useful and adapting them. It is possible to understand the basic principles and it will undoubtedly improve the quality of your life. It is worth looking into the bagua aspect of feng shui. Again, you don't need to go mad with it. Spend 20 minutes finding out where the rooms in your house are that relate to different aspects of your life – finances, relationships, etc. – and you may find the process revealing. It could be, for instance, that if you're consistently having financial problems, the 'finance area' of your house just happens to be your junk room!

One of the best books to explain the bagua well is *Creating Sacred Space with Feng Shui* by Karen Kingston. Also look at **www.firehorsefengshui.co.uk**.

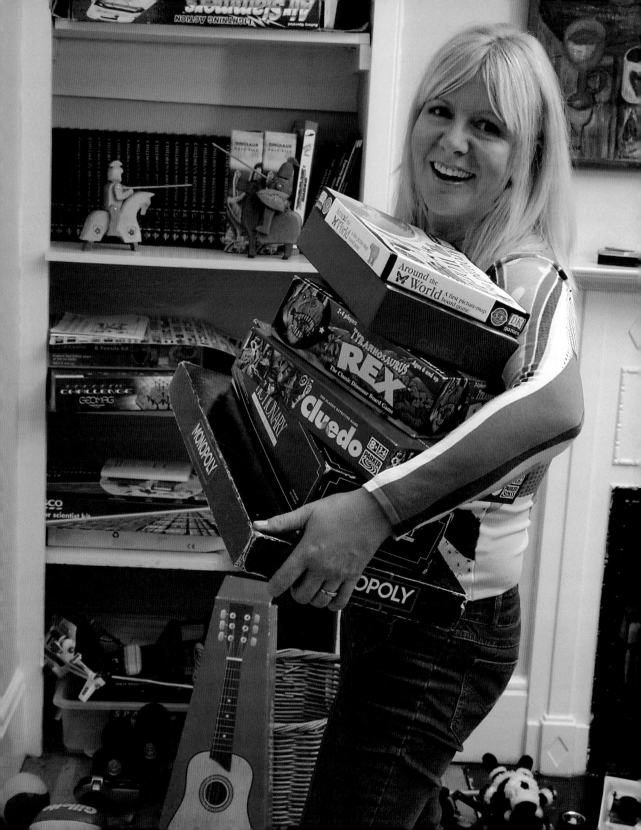

CLUTTER-CLEARING

When it comes to clearing your clutter, William Morris's words are a superb rule of thumb, and I try to go one step further with 'If it isn't beautiful, or I haven't used or worn it for six months, out it goes!' If you accept the basic feng shui principle that everything has an energy, it's clear that clutter and anything you don't need is just 'stuck' energy, and it will weigh you down, physically and emotionally. Maybe a lot of your possessions are nostalgic and remind you of a happy time in your life – well, get rid of them and you can pave the way for even happier times.

The problem often can be finding the courage to just let things go. We sometimes seem to have an instinctive urge to cling on to emotional baggage. Top feng shui expert Davina Makail calls these areas 'clutter blind spots'. When she came to help 'sort me out', we jumped in at the deep end, ransacking my endless cupboards and drawers, looking at every single item and she made me answer these questions:

- Do I really love this object?
- Does it enhance my life?
- Do I use it?
- Is it time to let it go?

First was my wardrobe, and out went anything that just didn't fit any more. After a little while I got into the swing of it. Two bin bags down the line it got to the point where she would simply hold an item up and look at me with a wry smile, and I would snatch it from her grasp, pushing it into the bin bag before she even had a chance to speak. I was enjoying this!

'Have nothing in your home that you do not know to be useful or believe to be beautiful.' William Morris

Admittedly, it was slightly difficult when it came to some of my sparkly 1980s kit, but boy was it a buzz when I dumped it all in nine bin bags in a charity shop. We went on to look at everything in the house that we had time for in one day, and the buzz of the 'getting rid' process turned out to be as revitalising as my new junk-free home later proved to be.

Books

Will you ever read them again? If not, why are you keeping them? Davina explained that energetically they represent old knowledge and old ideas. The double whammy is you can clear them out and benefit someone else by giving them to charity.

Photographs

These represent past memories. Keep current ones on display. Get rid of photos of old relationships, as they'll hamper your new ones.

Gifts

Don't let the fact that something was a gift be a reason for compulsory attachment to something you don't want, no matter who gave it to you. The real gift was in the giving and the moment between you and the giver, and that can never be lost.

Kitchen

Most people have kitchen cupboards that are overflowing with equipment they'll never use. Some kitchen items really are redundant. No one really needs an electric can opener, do they? Sandwich makers are slightly pointless, and remember the old days when we used a grill to toast our bread? Have a good clear-out of what you no longer use.

With almost any item you come across you'll have to fight emotional attachment, and the little devil on your shoulder will always give you a good reason why you have to hang on to it – for example:

- 'It might come in useful one day.' If it hasn't in the last year or so, it's unlikely that it ever will.
- 'But this cost a fortune.' One of the worst. Knowing that you spent a lot of money on something you never use will depress you every time you look at it; 'eBaying' it or just giving it away to someone who needs it will give you back that lost energy.

Clearing your clutter, reducing your 'possessions' and simplifying your surroundings is one sure, but often forgotten, way to creating a healthy energising environment in your home. Only then can you start to live for today!

To book a consultation with Davina Mackail for space clearing, feng shui, or geopathic stress clearing, go to **www.mackail.co.uk**.

If you're keen on clearing your clutter but without the feng shui approach, another excellent clutter-clearing expert is Naomi Saunders. She came and helped me to set up a system for my messy office.

Her book is called *Simplify Your Life: Downsize and De-stress*. She agrees that you should sort everything into three piles – cherish, charity, chuck – and reminds us that we will always appreciate space more than junk.

Another excellent read is *Organizing for the Creative Person* by Dorothy Lehmkuhl, Dolores Lamping and Dolores Cotter Lamping. It highlights the fact that depending on your personality you may have to set up paperwork systems to suit you, which are totally different to those of your colleague or partner. As a visual and very untidy person, I need three or four big bins clearly labelled that I can just throw things into, while my husband, who has a slightly more organised mind, finds piles of paperwork in files and in-trays actually do get dealt with.

It's much easier to get motivated with someone's help, so if you don't want to hire a clutter-clearing expert, just ask a friend to help you. You can return the favour because even if your own space is full of clutter, it's usually easier to be objective about someone else's.

'Life is constantly changing and evolving and our homes are a reflection of this. We never own anything in life, we only have things for a while and then we must let them move on, allowing the space for new beginnings.' Davina Makail

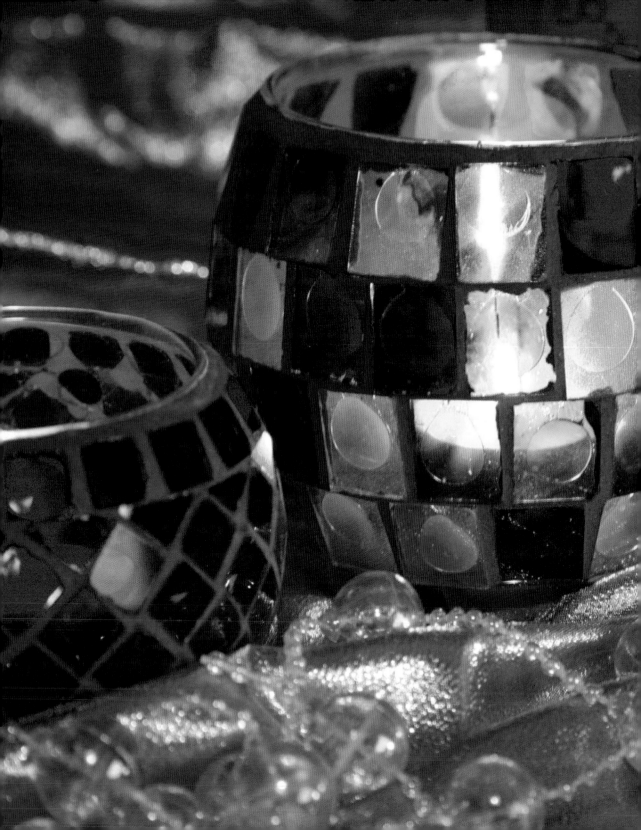

12 Lighting and colour

LIGHTING

'Wow, I love this room!'

Have you ever said that while house hunting or looking for a flat to rent? Why? 'It's so light. The sun just streams in here . . .' Maybe it's not even the room we love, but the light in the room. Light affects us in such an important way, and exposure, or lack of, to it plays a big part in the way we are able to work rest and play (see page 114). There's always been a natural God-given pattern of light supply to us, helping to regulate our body clocks in the most beneficial to way to us as a species. Being imperfect, though, we're going to want to mess with it of course, and party and work all night. Now I'm not suggesting that we go back to some pre-electric age where everything is done by the position of the sun – in fact more the opposite. Let's realise the potential of light, and how we can manipulate it to fantastic effect, to enhance our feelings moods and creativity in work and play, and ultimately our health and well-being.

Many years ago I moved into a new house and quickly allocated one of the rooms as my office. The desk was promptly installed. Slowly the paperwork began to pile up, and when I did make an effort, I found myself having to move everything on to the kitchen table before I could work. How many of us have done that?

Truth is, I was never going to get anything done in that office because the room's light made it a room to 'chill out' in.

After that quick learning curve, I found I began to enjoy being in rooms that had previously just 'drained my energy' or weren't enabling me to achieve what I wanted to, simply by changing the lighting. Let's face it: you wouldn't want white strip lights in your bedroom, even though they're pretty good for Dad's workshop. Energy-saving is a key issue with all of us now, and even with the onslaught of the rather depressing energy-saving bulb (see page 59), there are still ways you can achieve a good balance between this and getting the right light in your home to make you feel and work great.

Colour plays an equally important part too, and light can only enhance colour tones that already exist. You can improve a bad room colour with lighting, but sometimes you just need to get out the paint brush first.

LIGHT AS THERAPY

I go on at length about light as therapy in my first book *Imperfectly Natural Woman* but my enthusiasm for it has not waned.

Daylight is crucial for our well-being. Light intensity is measured in lux and on a summer's day we may have up to 16 hours of daylight at 100,000 lux, but that can drop to less than 5,000 on a gloomy day. It's well documented that you don't have to be suffering from seasonal affective disorder (SAD – see www.sad.co.uk) to feel lethargic and have a touch of the winter blues in the winter months. It may surprise you to know that indoor lighting rarely exceeds 500 lux, so you can see why we feel deficient in those sunny 'feel-good' hormones.

People suffering from depression can be greatly helped by a light treatment. I know it seems fairly artificial rather than natural for me to be encouraging you to plug in yet another appliance, but the good news is you don't need to have bright light on for very long to feel amazing benefits. Just 15 or 20 minutes will sort out your melatonin levels and leaving you with a spring in your step.

Light therapy works by simulating the light found in natural daylight to re-set our circadian rhythm. You can get a whole range of light therapy boxes and bulbs from www.wholistic research.com.

If you want a truly portable lightbox, the Litebook Elite (see www.litebook.com) is fantastic. I used mine in transit at Hong Kong Airport when I was trying to adjust my poor body clock after flying from Sydney (don't ask about carbon offsetting!). It really lifted my exhaustion and helped me get on the next morning flight feeling a bit more human.

It was previously thought that full spectrum light is what is required to treat light deficiency disorders, but new research shows that low-intensity blue light is twice as effective as other white light therapy treatments. Apollo Health (www.apollo-health.co.uk) have now used LEDs to produce the specific exclusive clinically proven 'bluewave technology', which offers quicker treatment times. Their Golite M2 weighs less than 11b, so it's very portable, and it has a built-in treatment timer and alarm clock.

Light up your workplace

The Health & Safety Executive found that work-related stress is the second most common type of occupational ill health, after muscular-skeletal or back problems, and 6.5 million sick days are taken in the UK because of stress. If you feel stressed or low, it's possible that the lighting in your workplace is a contributory factor. If you can't persuade the boss to change the infrastructure, at least take in your own lightbox – and it goes without saying grab the desk near the window for maximum efficiency.

Daylight alarm clocks

Remember that cockerel alarm clock you had when you were a child? Bin it! In an ideal world we'd all go to sleep earlier and rise with the sun, but that's not practical for most of us. At least if you have to have an alarm clock, choose one that wakes you gently. I use the Bodyclock Sunray, which has a thirty-minute 'sunrise' that wakes you gently, and if the light hasn't woken you at the requested time it makes a gentle peeping sound. It's not strictly light as therapy but it's certainly a therapeutic way to be awoken from a deep sleep. It costs approximately £60 from www.wholistic research.com. There's also the excellent Daybreak sunrise-sunset simulator, which works with the bedside lamp you already have, available from www.sad.co.uk.

One of my forum members on www.imperfectlynatural.com has an innovative idea. She says: 'I have a daylight simulator bulb on my bedside lamp, with a timer which switches it on approximately half an hour before the alarm clock rings, so it helps me to wake up gently to 'natural' light without needing to invest in a daylight alarm clock.' What a brilliant money-saving suggestion!

Himalayan salt lamps

Himalayan salt is a real treat, whether used as a detoxifying bath or taken internally (yes, you can make fish and chips healthy!). It contains at least 84 mineral elements that the body needs and is a natural antihistamine. How is that relevant to light? Well, you can buy Himalayan salt lamps, which are said to help ionise the air and improve sleep quality, and if nothing else they give off a lovely warm orange glow. Amazing Health (amazinghealth.co.uk) also sell a rare white Himalayan salt lamp that can be used with different colour bulbs.

I also love the Himalayan tea light. You just pop a tea light candle into it and it glows beautifully. Available from www.saltshack.co.uk and www.kudorrocksalt.co.uk.

COLOUR

On my Imperfectly Natural travels I met an inspiring woman called Juliet Standish, who offers a personalised colour consultancy service (www.colourconsultancy.co.uk). She says that even for yourself on a daily basis the colours you wear will affect your moods. It's thought that blue calms the nerves but could also increase weight gain. Its opposite colour, yellow, is said to promote energy and exercise so can help weight loss. I'm off to find a yellow jumpsuit!

Juliet explained to me the different effects choice of colour can have:

'Colours affect our moods and our emotions. They can inspire us or calm us, as well as providing a healing environment. Learning how to use colour in your home with decorations, furnishings, clothes and even colourful food can therefore help you to create the balance you need to lead a healthy and happy life.'

Some great books to read include *Colour Healing* by Lilian Verner-Bonds and *The Beginner's Guide to Colour Psychology* by Angela Wright.

It's incredible how too much of one colour can affect its occupants. If you think of an all-white ward in a hospital you can imagine how much more pleasant and healing it would feel if the pristine white were broken up with some bunches of lavender-pink flowers and some healthy green plants. Therapy rooms are often painted all white, but the therapist who is tuned in will have plants and perhaps even a spotlight, which can take different-coloured gels to harness the therapeutic effects of being bathed in coloured light.

So how do you go about selecting the right colours and shades to suit your home? First, I try to define each room, what I want to achieve in it, what colours and decorations would promote those aims, and how light would complement and enhance that.

Hallway

This gives the first impression of your house when entering, and the first thing you see when you arrive home from work. What do you want to feel? Maybe your workplace is hectic and you want to be relaxed when you open the front door with light pastels and minimalism. I want to be welcomed to something that loves and inspires me! I don't need detailed light, and I don't want to read. Because my hallway is fairly low on natural light, bright artwork beautifully lit with very imperfect low-voltage halogens will entice me in with a smile. I use a string of decorative LEDs to lift a dull corner too. Colourwise, Juliet says that white will expand a narrow hall, green indicates a harmonious home and pink suggests warmth within. Red is an inviting colour while yellow suggests a stimulating environment.

Living room

This should have a relaxed feel. My lighting is the old-style centre of the ceiling with a few lamps dotted around. I've used a mix of energy-saving and tungsten bulbs to avoid that death-white feel. (For lots more on energy-saving light bulbs and my personal view that

they're actually not all they're cracked up to be in terms of health and the environment, see page 59.)

The room also works well with the table lamps on their own. Colour-wise, blue soothes the nervous system (avoid very dark blue, which can be depressing to some) and also combines well with the balancing energy of green. Warm, dark colours can be very inviting and cosy. White is expansive and allows colour expression through curtains, cushions, pictures, etc. Yellow puts people in a good mood and beige or creams can be used but they need breaking up with vibrant touches of colour.

Kitchen and dining room

These are probably the heart of the family. Orange stimulates the appetite, particularly if combined with red, and it can also encourage communication and good health. However, if there are overeating disorders in the house, peaches or corals should be used instead in the dining area. To encourage gathering and sociability, choose warm shades of red, although not advisable for high blood pressure! Use gold accessories in the dining room to enhance a feeling of well-being among your guests. Green is the colour of balance and harmony and is therefore a good colour for any family room, and yellow wonderful for creativity and efficiency, which is great for a kitchen. Avoid blue, as it's too relaxing in a bustling kitchen. Strong working lights that are still 'friendly' are the order of the day here, and I can only achieve this with halogens. For dining, don't forget candles. Make sure you buy

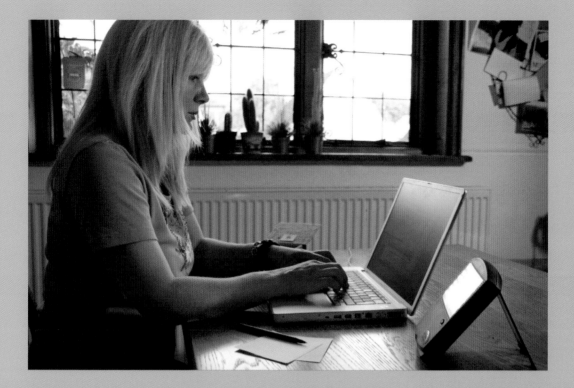

natural candles, though – I love the pure beeswax ones from **www.indigoessences. co.uk** and **www.brighterblessings.com**, who make gorgeous gift sets. You can also get halved coconuts with a wick added to create the most gorgeous-smelling candles.

Study

I find I need so much light here that I've taken to using full spectrum units, or light boxes (see chapter on light therapy) especially if I'm working late at night trying frantically to finish things like the book you're reading now! The rest of the time it's a sunny room, which is why I chose it as an office, but on a miserable day,

a brightish energy-saving light bulb works well. Juliet says, 'The home office is often an area where stimulation is needed for heightening the intellect so choose white, or yellow perhaps combined with blue. Avoid browns, greys and too much black, which could make you feel tired and non-productive.'

Remember light is especially important in the office; see also page 140 for information about the role of plants as therapy.

Children's rooms

These should have soothing colours for sleep to create a balance in children's emotional and physical well-being, while stimulating colours

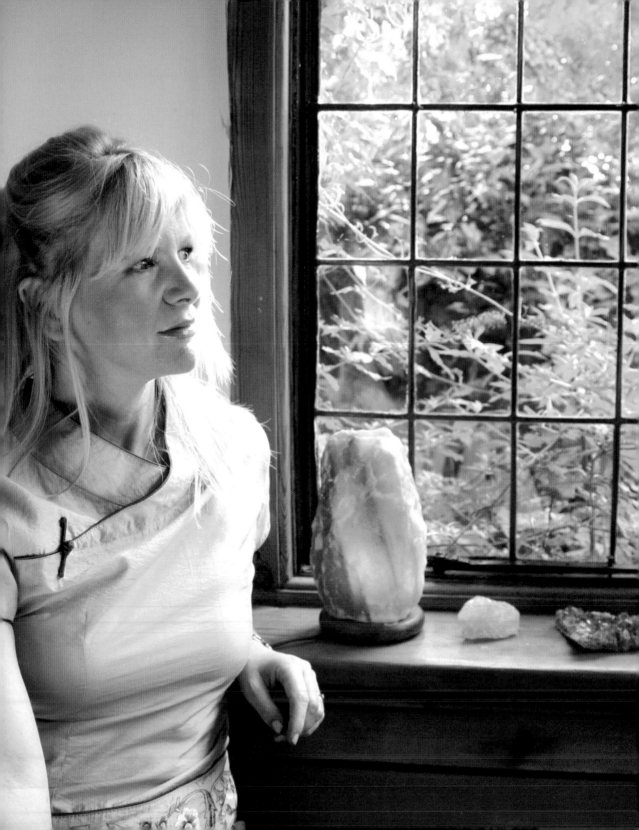

should be used in playrooms. If the bedroom combines as playroom, make it predominantly conducive to sleep. Lighting-wise, I find it's only relevant at tuck-in time, so almost anything goes.

Bedrooms

These should be places of retreat and lashings of romance, I hope, so soft hues are best. Yellow is much too stimulating to sleep in. Violet or indigo will make small bedrooms look larger and help you through periods of emotional trauma. Some red is great for creating sensuality, but in moderation, so pink, being a tint of red, is a great alternative. I use candles (don't fall asleep with them lit) and even fairy lights. Philips (www.philips.com) do an innovative LED light with a touch-sensitive remote control to enable you to change the colour depending on your 'bedroom mood'.

Nice bedside lamps – definitely not halogens – with transformers (see page 137 [Electro Protection]) are a must when you're doing that 'married couples' thing and reading a Jackie Collins novel, rather than having a night of passion.

Bathrooms

These need a relaxing colour. Blues are often chosen because of the resemblance of the sea. White will add light, and all coral colours add warmth because of the colour combination of red and yellow.

Stores, cupboards, utilities, etc.

For lighting in most other rooms, I'm reluctantly happy with energy-savers.

COLOUR ACCESSORIES

Remember that for therapeutic colour, you don't have to redecorate (but if you are going to, please consider eco paints – see page 124). It's great to use splashes of colour in your accessories. Different-coloured throws and cushions can completely change the feel of any room and cover up furniture that's looking a bit shabby.

Look to other cultures for their rich, colourful fabrics and choose fairly traded sustainable goods. Natural Collection (www.naturalcollection.com) has a sumptuous Bedouin range of vibrant hand-stitched bright cotton throws and cushions with starbursts of tiny mirrors and sequins. They're Fairtrade and made by a group in India who support a children's charity. If you're patient enough to sew, it's long gone out of fashion but cutting up bits of fabric and making your own hotchpotch patchwork quilt is a wonderful thing to do and to hand down to your children.

Imperfectly natural home Q&A

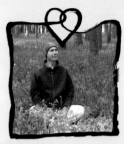

Martin Jones
Healer, cranio sacral therapist and founder of holographic breathing
www.holographic-breathing.com

Describe your home.
I live on my own and in a 72' x 12' barge on the Grand Union Canal.

How would you describe your interior 'style' and furnishings? I designed the shell and fitted it out with solid ash floors ceilings and walls; it's all open plan.

What does your home mean to you? A place to relax in nature, it's half a mile to the nearest road or house, and the countryside and wildlife is beautiful.

Have you attempted any eco DIY or modifications for a greener home? E.g. solar panels, eco paints, wind turbines etc. Was it worth it financially? The shell has foam spray insulation and large triple glazed windows, so there is almost no heat loss. The heating is a wood and coal burning stove, which gives a lovely feel to things. All the electricity is from solar panels and wind generation, and the water is from rainwater harvesting.

How would your home rate for energy-efficiency? What have you done to reduce energy usage? When you buy new appliances, do you consider the energy-efficiency? I think the energy rating is good and my only appliances are a gas hob, a stereo and radio.

What ideas do you have for 'water saving'? Install rainwater harvesting, there's loads of water.

How 'eco' is your furniture, floorings and furnishings? It's all wood and the bed's organic wool.

What cleaning/laundry/stain-removing products do you use? I use an eco powder and washing balls for the laundry, a little bit of eco washing up liquid, and a broom.

If you could buy any one 'eco' gadget or item for your home, inside or out, what would it be? A new wind generator.

What kind of cookware do you use? Non-stick/cast iron? It's mainly stainless steel.

What's your best tip for getting your fridge and larder stocked with healthy food? I don't have a fridge. I'm a vegan and eat mainly raw food. I just buy and eat, everything is fresh and tastes lovely.

www.rawreform.co.uk is a great website for fantastic salads, juices and tips.

What about composting? Yes, I have a compost.

What do you regularly recycle? How? (E.g. door collection) I go to the recycle depot, it's mainly bottles

What are your 'alternative' pet tips? No pets, but herons, kingfishers, cormorants and terns all fish around the boat. Foxes and badgers have their dens close by and there were two swallows hovering around inside the boat the other day.

What are your views on the possible dangers of electro 'smog'/wifi/emfs etc.? Have you taken any protective measures? I wear a small silver shield.

Do you know your carbon footprint and do you care about it? (Be honest!) The earth and nature is very much part of my life, and I feel that earth's energy and the heavenly energies are reflected in us, what we do to the earth we do to ourselves.

How green are you – lime/olive? I guess I'm olive.

Do you have an imperfectly natural guilty secret? I have a small van I truck around in – I think that is most of my carbon footprint.

What would your dream home be like? I would quite like to have a yacht and to go south in the winter.

What are your top three tips for a naturally healthy home?
1. Go for walks in the countryside and enjoy nature.
2. Try learning to talk with the earth; she is an alive and wondrous being. Once you start reconnecting and making friends, it is automatic to want things that are in harmony with her and yourself. Holographic breathing is a meditative, self-healing system. One of the things we can experience with this system is our connection to the earth and the higher energies, and their reflection within us. There is a free online audio lecture at **www.holographic-breathing.com**.

13 Moving home

DOWNSHIFTING

'For fast-acting relief try slowing down.' Lily Tomlin, actress, comedian

I used to think the word 'downshifting' meant moving to a smaller property, perhaps because the children had left home or you'd got divorced and suddenly found that a one-bedroom apartment was sufficient. Actually it's about much more than just moving 'down' out of financial necessity; it's about making a conscious lifestyle choice which can often result in a happier, more relaxed, greener and, yes, more financially viable way of life.

There's a great website, www.downshiftingweek.com, which is all about such an initiative. You can download a free downshifting planner and there's a free e-book called 'Slow Down and Green Up'.

MOVING

But whether you're moving house to downsize or indeed go up in the world, you'll need a few tips on moving house

Boxes become a big part of your life when you're about to move house and all I can suggest is that you beg and borrow boxes and containers from friends. You'll almost certainly need to buy

some, but they're extremely expensive and a huge waste of resources if they're not re-used.

Fortunately several removal firms now offer recycled boxes that can be used over and over, and they'll collect them from you after you've unpacked.

It goes without saying that you should read again about clutter clearing (page 108) – don't move house taking all your old clutter with you! It's a great time to get rid of unwanted stuff, so start the sorting out as far in advance as you can, to allow you time to sell the unwanted items or give them away (see page 108).

In many houses the so-called box room is exactly that; for years on end it simply contains boxes. If you store boxes in a spare room or attic, they probably won't get opened until you move again.

Make sure you pack items pertaining to certain rooms together, and always, but always, label the box with the name of the room it needs to be positioned in at your new home.

AVOIDING STRESS

Now I am going to have to get cosmic again, but before you write it all off as nonsense just stop and think how evocative your memories are of your childhood home. I'd guess that you can still see in great detail every room in the

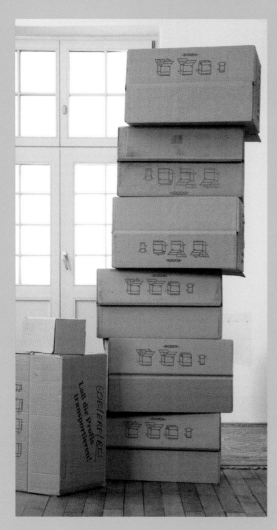

'When humans participate in ceremony, they enter a sacred space. Everything outside of that space shrivels in importance. Time takes on a different dimension. Emotions flow more freely. The bodies of participants become filled with the energy of life, and this energy reaches out and blesses the creation around them. All is made new; everything becomes sacred.' Sun Bear

desired new house or the beginning of living with a partner for the first time. A good way to dispel some of the stress is to ensure that your last thoughts of the home you leave are happy.

When the last vanload of possessions is on its way, clean your house (obviously you'll need to leave out the cleaning materials). I know it sounds slightly bizarre to be cleaning up for someone else, but if you believe in karma you'll appreciate that someone else will do it for you too.

Walk into every room in your home, and open your arms and say thank you – remember happy times and leave behind a good energy. You could even hold a little goodbye ceremony to 'let the house go' and help you take happy memories away with you.

house you grew up in and whenever you're reminded of certain smells it will take you back there. I'd guess you can remember the first home you owned too. There's no doubt our memories and our hopes and dreams are all entwined with our accommodation.

Because we form such an emotional attachment to our homes, moving can be a hugely traumatic experience, even if it's a much-

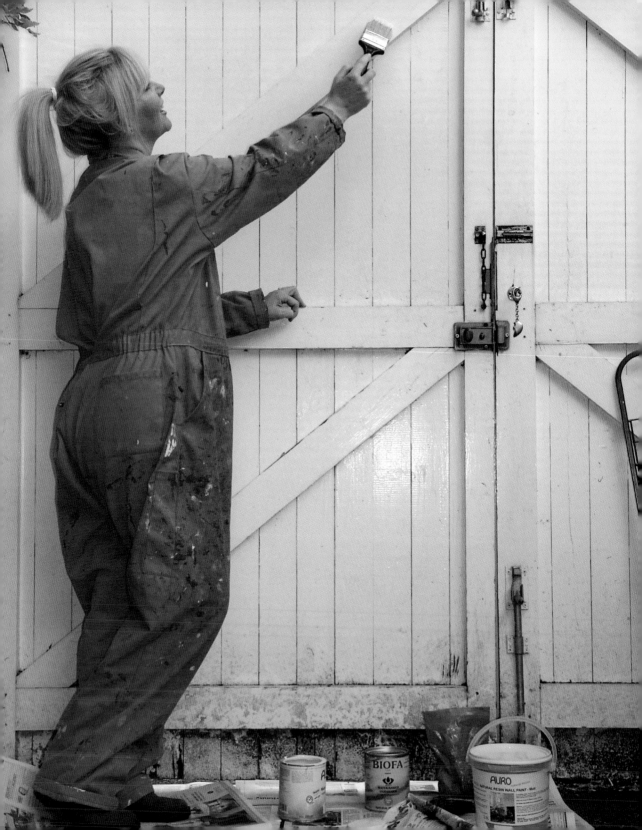

14 DIY and materials

'The fellow that owns his own home is always just coming out of a hardware store.' Kin Hubbard, journalist

Now DIY's enough of a minefield without me sticking my oar in, but all the same in this section I've investigated most of our popular weekend DIY pursuits, and hopefully in keeping with my favourite catchphrase, I've found an Imperfectly Natural alternative to many of them.

It has to be said – generalising wildly here – this is a domain somewhat favoured by you blokes, but in true macho style, admit it, you sometimes aren't quite so conscious as us girls when it comes to the harmful-chemicals-in-our-homes predicament. Often it's just a case of back from the DIY store, 'This stuff is the bizniz – gets the job done!' and not taking much notice of tins festooned with black crosses and skull and crossbones insignias (apologies to all eco men). Admittedly, you're not slapping that epoxy glue, plumber's resin or woodworm treatment on your faces (though some of the ingredients are similar), but the point is that all this stuff we use – resins, building materials, paints, solvents – remain in our environment long after the work is done, still 'off-gassing' and still affecting us on a daily basis.

In true imperfect style, sometimes a dose of high-strength sulphuric acid is the only thing that will clear a blocked drain, but the fact remains that thousands of those tins you buy from DIY stores are going to contain things you don't want to be too up close and personal with, and for so many products there are some great alternatives.

ECO-CONFUSION

One thing to bear in mind, though, is that the world of eco alternatives in this area is a minefield. One company's definition of an eco-friendly product may differ from another's.

Take, for example, pigments in paints. Some will argue that using natural pigments is not eco-friendly because it can involve quarrying, which is damaging to the environment, and they will therefore use chemical ones. Others will argue that natural pigments are less toxic, so therefore should be the choice for using on your walls, despite possible environmental damage in obtaining them.

Many 'nasties' in building and other products are 'hidden' by being inserted at earlier stages of the manufacturing process and thus by legal wizardry avoiding being named on the tin. Of course not all manufacturers are unscrupulous, and all must be within the law, but the green movement is a bandwagon for much big business, and being able to insert the words 'natural' on your product is, in the current climate, a big plus for potential sales.

There's also the added worry that 'natural' doesn't necessarily mean 'not poisonous'. So unless you want to make it a career, it's impossible to get your choices absolutely right. Being Imperfectly Natural really is your get-out clause here. When sourcing products and materials, I tend to look for small independent pioneer-style manufacturers, people whose hearts seem in the right place.

Always look for the simple common-sense solution, and usually by default you'll end up with an eco-friendly one. Also, with any work I need done in the house, a good rule of thumb that I always try to stick to is 'renew and repair before you replace'. I'll get a handyman or someone useful to fix that broken door panel, rather than schlock down to the local mega DIY place for a new one that will not only cost me more but will perhaps be impregnated in preservative and formaldehyde.

There are now some great sources of eco building products. Try **www.natural-building.co.uk**, **www.oldhousestore.co.uk**, **www.greenshop.co.uk** or **www.ecomerchant.co.uk**.

Happy DIY! Or in my Imperfectly Natural style, I think I'll just let hubby get on with it . . .

PAINTS

Paints are a big issue, and I know of people who have undesirable levels of toxins in their systems as a result of working with them. There are loads of types, including epoxy urea-formaldehyde, latex, and oil-based. Lead in paint is only usually an issue with older buildings. If you do have old leaded paint and it's still in relatively sound condition, it can be simpler to not 'wake the sleeping giant' by merely painting over it, but if you want it eliminated altogether you'll need to get professional advice before scraping it off. Paints can contain petrochemical solvents, fungicides – all manner of things that can contribute to conditions such as asthma, allergies and sick building syndrome. Even arsenic was used as a pigment for many years.

I would definitely not want to be breathing that lot in, and unless you're in a position to move out for a week when you decorate, I would opt for organic and eco paints. Some eco paints on the market are more eco than others and, as I've already mentioned, everyone has a different definition of the word eco. Many eco paints will still contain solvents and VOCs, but at significantly reduced levels. Ecos Organic Paints (**www.ecospaints.com**) make a wide range of paints, sealants, stains and glues, free of solvents and VOCs; they also make electrical radiation protection paint (see page 138). Osmo (**www.osmouk.com**) have a very good reputation for a strong long-lasting product, after all, it's not very green if you have to paint your walls again too soon. I also like Auro (**www.auro.co.uk**), who do a lovely range of natural colours, and Biofa paints from **www.villanatura.co.uk**.

PAINT STRIPPERS

These are scary, and the fumes alone can knock you for six. They can contain harsh solvents, a common one being dichloromethane, a highly toxic known carcinogen. Opt for removing paint with heat (be careful) or try an eco alternative such as Homestrip from www.greenbuildingstore.co.uk. A real eco alternative is to try pasting on mineral washing soda, available in hardware stores and some supermarkets (leave it on for about six hours, and try to not let it dry out).

WALLPAPER

Most wallpapers contain solvents, but you can get eco wallpaper such as the beautiful Harry's Garden design available from www.ecocentric.co.uk. The range is printed in the UK on chlorine-free paper sourced from managed forests, the inks are water-based with no use of hazardous solvents and any waste from edge trimmings is recycled.

Fortunately you can also buy eco wallpaper glue free from fungicides, preservatives and synthetic resins from www.urbanliving.co.uk.

WOOD PRESERVATIVES

Many wood preservatives contain biocides which, to cut a long story short, and despite attempts to make them safe, are designed basically to kill living things. Go for an eco option such as Osmo Wood protector from www.lowimpact.org.

You can buy water-thinnable, solvent-free finishes that don't contain biocides and are therefore great for cots and children's toys from Auro (www.auro.co.uk). They also sell a range of floor finishes to keep wood looking close to its original colour and do not 'fire' or darken the wood as oil-based finishes do, as well as interior and exterior wood finishes and wood stains that are solvent-free.

CARPETS

Stained mucky carpets have become the bane of my life since having children and if I owned the house I'm now living in, I'd rip them up in every room. As well as emitting yet more VOCs in your home, most carpets are laced with all manner of potentially toxic substances including petroleum by-products, latex, mothproofing chemicals (naphthalene), antimicrobial treatments, fire retardants containing PBDEs (which can cause thyroid and immune system damage) and other chemicals that I'd prefer to avoid. It's even more of an issue with older carpets, as they may contain chemicals that have since been banned.

Ever wondered what that nice smell is on new carpets? Well, it's very often a substance worryingly called 4-PC, which has been associated with eye, nose and upper respiratory problems, and will happily spend an age leaching into your room long after you've forgotten about it (another little bit of my 'toxin accumulation' theory).

I've already suggested ways of cleaning the carpet (see page 15), and I also suggest you consider flooring alternatives (see below), but the good news is that if you want carpets you can now get some more 'natural options' that are infinitely preferable to the synthetic fibres that most regular carpets are made from.

For starters, avoid the traditional foam or latex backing and go for one that has jute or wool backing. For the actual carpet, opt for wool that is unbleached and coloured with natural plant-based dyes. Bear in mind that regular wool carpets are often treated with pesticides. You can also now get carpet tiles, which make replacement much easier and cheaper – see **www.heuga.com**.

OTHER FLOORING

Other options for natural flooring that are becoming more popular are seagrass, which is made by flooding the plant with seawater before harvesting; sisal, which is made from the leaves of the Agave sisalana plant; and jute and coir. They are all very hard wearing, but not always as soft underfoot as you might be used to after the shagpile carpet. Whichever you use, check what it's treated with, and consider the adhesives used in the laying process too.

If you can afford it, for a kitchen or conservatory, terracotta or marble tiles can look fantastic, are really easy to clean and will reduce dust mites and allergens. Fired Earth make a wonderful range of floor tiles as well as other natural floorings – not cheap, but fab.

Old-style linoleum is definitely hip again. It's usually made from plants such as linseed or jute – though make sure it's proper lino from natural resins, and not just PVC sheeting – and it's long-lasting. It can be put to good re-use as an underlay when you've decided you no longer want a zebra-skin-patterned bathroom!

Bamboo is increasing in popularity. It's very eco-friendly and makes a great floor that is harder than oak, and it's half the cost. Most of it has travelled quite a bit to get to us, so it doesn't score brilliantly on the air miles front, but it is very sustainable – a 60-foot-high plant can grow in a few months, compared to 50 years for an oak tree the same height. Well worth looking into are **www.pandaflooring.co.uk** and **www.zenflooring.co.uk**.

If you're splashing out on flooring, look into recycled wood. The obvious environmental benefits aside, it looks amazing. Hardwoods look mature and rustic, often have a denser grain and are full of character. It's a kind of investment too, as it increases the saleable value of your pad. Many flooring suppliers sell 'reclaimed' wood alongside their new stock. Check out **www.chauncey.co.uk** and **www.priorsrec.co.uk** (also great for reclaimed doors and tiles). Wood that has been responsibly and ecologically sourced should have the FSC stamp of approval. Christina Meyer (**www.christinameyer.com**) also produces a good range.

Check out timber laminate floors made from recycled timber or timber from a well managed, preferably UK, FSC-approved source. Amtico (**www.amtico.co.uk**) and Karndean (**www.karndean.co.uk**) make very hardwearing PVC-free versions.

Marmoleum made by Forbo (**www.forbo-flooring.co.uk**) is a great versatile choice for hard flooring. Made from linseed oil and chalk, it comes in a huge range of colours, and is warm underfoot, waterproof and completely antistatic – a good choice for bathrooms or kitchens.

You can also get cork tiles, which keep a highly sustainable industry in Portugal going, but check that they are not sealed with PVC.

See also **www.naturalflooring.net** and **www.alternativeflooring.co.uk**.

If though, like me, you're not currently in the business of new flooring, odds on there's a great softwood floor under that stinky old carpet just waiting to be sanded. If I weren't renting at the moment, I'd rip the carpets up, pack them off with their millions of unpaying dust-mite guests, and just sand and treat the floorboards with an organic finish.

Try it out in one small room first, and hopefully the results will encourage you to go for a bigger room. Use a water-based sealant or an eco floor finish such as Hardwax Oil from Osmouk or Auro as above.

If you can't get the wood to look good, just painting floors even in white looks great too; the unevenness and cragginess of the floor just adds to the effect. Bear in mind, though, that pulling up the carpets can make your house feel more draughty.

WOODEN FIXTURES AND FITTINGS

I know the likes of Changing Rooms would have you believe that MDF (and a stapler) is the answer to everything, but I hate it. It's flimsy, ungrounding and often impregnated with formaldehyde. This is more of a risk when you're working with the stuff, but even if you're not it will spend its life leaching nasties into your surroundings, albeit at low levels. I'm not saying rip all your MDF out – that could release more chemicals into your surroundings than just leaving it be – but don't use it new, out of choice. If you have to use some sort of panelling, chipboard fares slightly better, and some makes avoid formaldehyde by using polyurethane instead. Panelvent (see **www.panelagency.co.uk**), manufactured from wood chips and forest thinnings, has low formaldehyde emissions in use and low embodied energy in manufacture, so is a more eco-friendly option.

Again, I will always try to go for old and recycled or reclaimed. If you're replacing, for example, your kitchen cupboard doors, you'll be amazed how individual your kitchen will look with recycled materials. Try **www.freecycle.org.uk**, and **www.salvo.co.uk** is a great website for all things reclaimed, from fireplaces to furnishings.

ROT AND DAMP

Many surveyors would have you flinging your hands to your faces at the very mention of the

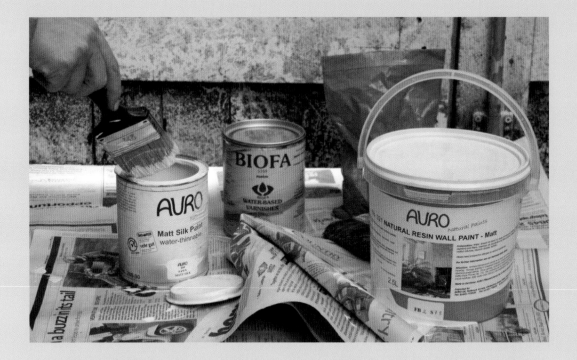

words 'rot' and 'damp', but the main thing here is don't panic!

Top eco-surveyor Mary Craig will always look for the simple solution first. She says:
Most surveys of old buildings and even some new ones mention the word 'damp' and recommend getting someone else in to tell you if it's a problem or not. There are plenty of companies out there who will carry out a free survey then recommend work that could result in you introducing any amount of unnecessary chemicals into your building to treat a problem that isn't a problem. Damp can cause physical and unsightly damage and it can support insect attack in timber – in extreme cases this can lead to structural damage of the building. It can also lead to rots and moulds forming, which can be hazardous to your health, especially if you are asthmatic.

But treatment of these 'symptoms' by dosing the area with a liberal amount of fungicide or pesticide is a completely pointless exercise if you don't sort the cause out. Water is either coming into the building or from the air in the form of condensation. Often you can find the cause yourself. Look for leaks from gutters or pipes (guttering simply clogged with leaves is one of the biggest causes of damp problems); check no one has blocked under-floor ventilation. Is there a soil level for your flower beds that has accidentally risen to above the damp proof course? Perhaps you have a pipe leak inside the house. Read your water meter, then don't use any water for a few hours or overnight, and see if the reading has changed. If so, you'll know you have a leak probably from pipe work inside.

Sort the problem out, then dry the building by increasing the ventilation and heating. If you have a condensation problem, this is often cured by increasing the ventilation and heating up the air. It may be that you are on to a loser trying to sort out damp in the cellar, but just don't use it as your bedroom!

Also watch out for the specialists: you don't have to toe the line with allegedly expert advice, especially from someone who has a vested interest in getting you to spend money. In *Imperfectly Natural Woman* I wrote about how a £2,000 damp quote was rendered unnecessary by a simple £30 repair job.

There are non-chemical alternatives to treating rot such as Thermo Lignum's WARMAIR process (see **www.thermo lignum.com**), although these can be much more expensive.

DRAINS

If you don't want the harshness of caustic soda, use one of the methods described on page 20.

WOODWORM

Woodworm can bring buildings down, but just because you see the little holes, it doesn't mean the little critters are still resident. Tape some sheets of paper over the holes and leave them for a day or so. If no new little holes appear, you'll know they've long gone and you don't have a problem. More info on alternative treatments from Thermo Lignum (**www.thermolignum.com**), who offer a detailed process, not cheap but nevertheless chemical-free.

WIRING

For all the DIY gadget enthusiasts here (I don't mean electricity – don't touch that!), hard wire everything – your doorbell, your alarm system, and especially your internet – instead of using wi-fi, and if possible get back your coily lead analogue phones. Don't install anything that just adds to the electro-smog around your person (see also page 134 on electro-protection). While I'm on electro stuff, ditch your mains drill (if you're still using one) and get a rechargeable drill. The EMFs (see page 134) that fly off those old-style mains drills are definitely to be avoided.

WINDOWS

It's worth keeping an eye on old windows, as unmaintained sash windows can be the source of some serious draughts. If yours are old, consider if they can be repaired rather than replaced. It's cheaper, uses fewer resources and helps to keep alive traditional skills.

If you're replacing windows, get advice, and look at some excellent models of practice such as the excellent green buildings at Trelowarren Estate in Cornwall (**www.trelowarren.co.uk**).

15 Water

DRINKING WATER

Unless you're visiting countries where regular water supplies are suspect (in those cases, at least go for water in glass bottles), I just don't see water in plastic bottles as a healthy or green option (see page 39). Far better to get a filtration system for your mains supply. The initial outlay is a fraction of what you'd spend buying bottles over time, and you'll save your back not having to carry them about in packs of eight. I've installed a reverse osmosis under sink system (see page 40).

FLUORIDE

I've written extensively about this in my other books. Suffice to say I'm very glad that my reverse osmosis under sink system is getting rid of it before it gets into me!

CHLORINE

I don't like the smell of chlorine, and in swimming pools it makes my eyes go red and

'We never know the worth of water till the well is dry.' Thomas Fuller, preacher

sore, my hair dry and brittle and my skin itchy. Chlorine is basically an antibiotic, easily absorbed into skin, and many of us, especially those prone to eczema, are affected.

If you love swimming, look for an ozone pool (chlorine-free) or at the very least shower immediately after being exposed to it. At home (now your drinking water's sorted out with a reverse osmosis under sink unit!), here's a little solution I found for the bathroom: an Anti Chlorine Bath Filter Ball from **www.sensitive skincareco.com**. Because your blood flow increases when you are in a hot bath, your skin and hair will absorb chlorine more rapidly. You inhale it too, as the chlorine vaporises with the heat of the water. This ball doesn't absorb the chlorine: it just changes it into harmless zinc chloride. It's dead cheap; just hang it over the tap flow as you're filling the bath and that's it. It'll last for 300 baths. Fantastic – I love a simple solution! Also, if you like a shower, there's the APHF PC Slimline Chrome Shower Dechlorination Filter from **www.sensitiveskincareco.com**, a neat little unit that fits on to your shower head and does the same job.

SAVING WATER

One good result of the recent hosepipe ban is that it got people into the mindset of water saving. Garden centres were inundated with requests for water butts and devices for recycling water.

So what are the really important messages here? Well, it all comes down to attitude. I personally think a blanket ban on hosepipes is ridiculous and does nothing to change the real problem of water usage being unsustainable. What is needed is more awareness of the real depth of the problem, as well as lots more effective easy-to-source products that help us to achieve the aim of using less water.

Ultimately, the ideal is sophisticated systems that use water that's already been used. The term is 'grey water' and of course that's what should be used to flush our toilets and wash our cars. See page 151 for more on rainwater harvesting and eco home of the future (page 174).

TOILETS

The humble toilet accounts for a third of total domestic water consumption in the UK. You don't need me to remind you I'm sure that up to a third of the world's population has no clean running water, so of course it's a disgrace that we flush away up to three gallons of pure drinkable water after having a quick pee. A slogan came back into fashion, didn't it: 'If it's yellow, let it mellow', meaning of course don't bother to flush unless it's 'number twos', but for many people that's an alien concept.

If you're renovating and installing toilets, go for a dual flush system. It'll reduce water usage by 67 per cent, compared to a traditional toilet. When I went to Australia recently, I saw dual systems nearly everywhere.

For existing toilets, fit a Save a Flush, a simple 'pop in the cistern' bag of harmless crystals, which can save 2,000 litres of water per person per year, or a Hippo, which will save you even more. Both are free from www.thameswater.co.uk. Or go to www.hippo-the-watersaver.co.uk.

SHOWERS

We all love a bath, but when you get used to having showers, they're just as refreshing, maybe more so. A five-minute shower uses less than half the water a bath uses, saving over 300 litres of water a week. Fitting a flow restrictor on either a mains or power shower will give you an optimum flow (6 litres a minute) for water saving and a nice shower.

HOT WATER

Lastly, turn the thermostat down. You'll save energy and see it in your bills. An ideal setting for hot water is 60°C/140°F.

'The biggest waste of water in the country is when you spend half a pint and flush two gallons.' Prince Philip, Duke of Edinburgh

16 Something in the air

'I durst not laugh for fear of opening my lips and receiving the bad air.' William Shakespeare

It's a worrying fact that we're exposed to more pollution in our own homes than when we're outdoors. As I've been saying throughout this book, building materials, toxic chemicals in our cleaning and personal care products, smoking and using air fresheners all add up, not to mention the effects of electromagnetic frequencies (EMFs) (see page 134).

We also spend more time in our centrally heated 'sealed' triple-glazed energy-efficient homes and as a result, we're susceptible to more allergies, skin conditions, headaches, colds, viruses, respiratory problems, and just plain fatigue. Inadequate ventilation is a major cause of 'sick building syndrome' and central heating dries out the moist mucosa in your nose which is the defence against invading viruses. Problems are compounded in our offices, workplaces and even shopping centres. Air-conditioning units are breeding grounds for all manner of viruses, and electronic equipment and artificial lighting can contribute to headaches and fatigue.

At work, you can't always say what goes, but at home you can make a difference.

IS YOUR HOME SICK?

Just as your body does sometimes, your house probably needs a health check, especially if you've just moved in. It's not time-consuming or scary, and much of what you'll need to do as a result will be a simple fix. Odds on you've got no problems, but if you do a health check it will enable you to lay the foundations of your healthy home.

Sick building syndrome isn't just limited to offices and work places, even though it was those which seemed to get all the press when this issue was first unearthed. It's easy to find that you have been living in a sick building for ages and unaware of it, for the simple reason that your senses become so attuned that you don't really notice it. Common sick building problems stem from fungi, mould, damp, carbon monoxide, radon, as well as issues involving ley lines, geopathic stress and EMFs. These are often hidden, and can affect you in subtle ways; some can even be killers.

Air quality is ultra important. Leaks and damp can create mould, which releases into the air spores that affect your general health. Look for little black or orange spots on ceilings and walls (for damp treatment, see page 127). Carbon monoxide detectors are cheap and easily available. EMF detectors are easily available too (see page 136). If you want to

get really thorough, radon is something worth checking for. It occurs naturally and is a colourless odourless radioactive gas, harmful if it accumulates to high levels. In my beloved St Ives in Cornwall it's a very real issue but those in the know have made sure that their buildings are well ventilated, not sealed and triple glazed to within an inch of their lives. Radon detector kits are priced between £30–50, available from www.radon.co.uk.

Issues involving lead or asbestos in your environment will of course need to be dealt with professionally.

ELECTRO-PROTECTION

Sometimes a little knowledge can be a dangerous thing, so you'll be delighted to know I don't intend to pretend to be scientific enough to give you all the intimate details on electromagnetic frequencies (EMFs).

In short, 'electro-pollution' – chronic exposure to weak electric fields and radiations from a myriad sources such as cell phones and powerlines – can sometimes lead to serious ill health, including increased chance of cancer and brain tumours and the suppression of melatonin, which helps us to sleep soundly.

I believe it's one of the biggest health issues facing us today, and it's not rocket science to realise that our homes are full of all kinds of electro-pollution that could, to a greater or lesser extent, be having a detrimental effect on our health and well-being.

Electro smog, or e-smog, is a very apt description for this problem. It's rather like the notorious smogs that blighted London up until the middle of the 20th century, except they could actually be seen, prompting people to do something about it. Until a century ago, nature hadn't encountered the electromagnetic fields ('EMFs') of modern life, so we are not prepared for them by evolution. There have been many investigative programmes looking at the effects of the increasingly present e-smog, the results of which seem to range from 'no real health risk' to the 'silent killer of the 21st century'. You could certainly argue that we seem to be making ourselves guinea pigs in the biggest mass biological experiment of all time. Fact remains there's no proof that it isn't a risk, and personally I believe we would be prudent to err on the precautionary side.

Some people are affected by e-smog so badly that they can't live in certain areas near mobile phone masts or power lines. Some report headaches when using cellular phones and many people just notice a huge difference in their well-being when they get away from their usual environment – away from the electro-pollution of their city or office – and perhaps out into the countryside (though these days that's not immune either).

The most relaxing short breaks I've had are in buildings that are 'low tech'. When I stayed

'We must learn to balance the material wonders of technology with the spiritual demands of our human race.' John Naisbitt, author

at Magdalen Court in Somerset and the holistic education centre and community at Monkton Wyld in Devon (see www.themagdalenproject.org.uk and www.monktonwyldcourt.org) for short courses I experienced an overwhelming sense of well-being just from the lack of electronic equipment. (The stunning countryside and history steeped into the walls helped too!)

Of course it's not viable to give up our technological lifestyles. Most of us in the UK now own mobile phones, cordless telephones, wi-fi, computers, microwave ovens and an array of electronic equipment. Outside our windows there is more than likely to be a mobile phone transmitter nearby and although it's claimed that there is no proven health risk from exposure to mobile phones, mobile phone masts or TETRA transmitters (used for police communications), unfortunately most of the safety guidelines are based on the assumption that the only harmful effect of microwaves is that they will 'cook' you at high enough power levels. There is, however, much research including that by the US Environmental Protection Agency and the World Health Organisation indicating biological effects at levels well below those required for a thermal effect … So what are being concocted, in effect, are allegedly 'safe' levels of exposure as guidelines for us all, whereas the reality is that there is much disagreement as to where those levels should be set, as well as much variation in different countries as to how levels are measured and what really is a safe level of exposure. For more information, see Roger Coghill's articles at www.cogreslab.co.uk.

WHERE ARE THE EMFS IN YOUR HOME?

As well as the high-frequency radiation from transmitters and wi-fi, and electro-pollution caused by electronic equipment in your home as described above, rather worrying are the 'fields' created by seemingly innocent items in your house such as cordless phones. Unlike mobiles, which transmit unwanted radiation only when in use, the base stations of cordless phones are transmitting powerful signals 24 hours a day, desperately trying to seek out their little receiver friends dotted around your house.

It's been said that the radiation from cordless systems flying around our houses is 100 times more dangerous than that transmitted by mobiles. Alasdair Philips of Powerwatch, the independent consultants and lobbyists for safety protection from electromagnetic fields and co-author of The Powerwatch Handbook, says, 'Cordless phones are now the standard in most households, and, like mobile handsets, they emit microwave radiation – from both the base unit and the handset itself – that is alleged to cause brain tumours, breast cancer, dementia, DNA damage, concentration problems, memory loss, mood and behavioural changes and fertility problems.'

I know of someone whose pet dog spent a year chewing its leg in a kind of manic frustration. She then began to suffer from hormonal problems and insomnia, and noticed that she too was becoming aggressive. She had a consultation with a therapist at Integral Nutrition (www.integralnutrition.co.uk), who suggested that she tried unplugging the cordless base station for the phone system. When she did so, the poor animal breathed a sigh of relief, for a day, until she switched the phones back on. Almost instantly the dog returned to its manic ways. Sometimes animals can be so much more in tune than us. Happily it's old-style cord phones round her place now.

When we sleep our bodies are at their most vulnerable to attack from unseen emissions. If I, or anyone in my family, suffered from long-term sleep problems, the first question I would ask myself is, do I live near a police station that houses a TETRA transmitter or G3 transmitter (the new extra-powerful mobile phone transmitters)? To find the nearest to you, go to **www.sitefinder.radio.gov.uk**.

If the answer was yes, my two options would be to move or do something to protect myself. Practically, it's going to be the latter for most of us. We aren't about to go back to candlelight, or carrier pigeons instead of our mobile and cordless phones (though those ideas are not too bad per se), but if we want to avoid EMFs there are things we can do to really make a difference.

SHIELD YOURSELF

The first thing to do is find out if you've got a problem. It's easy to check your house for electro-pollution. Rent or buy electric and magnetic meters from Healthy House (**www.healthy-house.co.uk**). They're simple to operate, and you can run a 15-minute check and discover any possible problems. Healthy House also rent out at under £20 an A-COM meter, which will check your home environment for pulsed frequencies from modern communication equipment and microwave sources.

In true Imperfectly Natural style you don't have to absolutely eliminate everything electrical. I made a few changes (see below) to mine and the kids' bedrooms, ran my borrowed meter over the pillows and was amazed how much the EMF readings had reduced. Encouraged by this, I went the whole hog, making more changes around the house. Sadly no sooner did I hardwire my internet and ditch my digital phones than my neighbours (who obviously haven't read my books yet!) installed wi-fi, which then happily zapped its way through my walls. But don't let that put you off: make sure you get hold of a meter and check. You may not have a problem at all, so don't spend and protect unnecessarily. But if you do, there are some ways you can minimise the risk.

I've more or less come to the conclusion that in a domestic situation, EMFs are impossible to escape from completely. The most important time to protect yourself, though, is during sleep, as EMFs interfere with the delicate neurological balances and mechanisms necessary for your body to 'repair' itself each night. TVs, computers, radios – in fact anything that you plug in emits radiation that can affect your sleep patterns. So if you can find ways of protecting your sleeping environment, you can be protected for one-third of your whole life – that being the amount of time you spend kipping. First remember to switch off electrical items you don't need at the wall, especially those near your head. Also beware of mains cables running under your bed. If you need things that plug in, again don't have them right next to your head. Change your halogen bedside lamp for a standard one, because a transformer emits a ton of EMFs, and odds on, that's on the floor right under your head, Same with plug-in alarm clocks. If you can't tolerate an old-style 'wind up', make sure your clock has the transformer at the wall plug end, and not built in to the clock – that way it will be further away from you.

Net screens for your bed can be made from material rather like mosquito nets. An invisible metal fibre is woven into the material, creating a deflective barrier that can stop up to 90 per cent of high-frequency radiation getting to you. Take that, oh neighbour! The material isn't cheap, but the nets are simple and effective, and can also look rather pretty. You'll need to put one under your mattress as well. Take your laptop to bed and look for wi-fi reception to test it out. The material is available from **www.healthy-house.co.uk**.

Roger Coghill, a leading expert in this field, is now manufacturing a food supplement called Asphalia. It is based on the plant version of the powerful brain hormone melatonin, which normally organises our sleep patterns, keeps us from ageing, and protects us against free radical damage. It's thought to protect against electro-smog too. **www.asphalia.co.uk**

GEOPATHIC STRESS NEUTRALISERS

Healthy house consultant Davina Mackail (see page 108) explains the problem of geopathic stress:

Very often I meet clients with allergies, asthma, immune deficiency diseases; headaches; tiredness; irritability and more serious diseases such as cancer. Often the cause of these issues can be traced back to environmental issues, chemical toxins, electromagnetic pollution and geopathic stress.

Geo (earth) pathic (disease) stress (GS) is a distorted electromagnetic field of the earth. The earth resonates with an electromagnetic frequency (EMF) of 7.83 Hz, which is identical to the alpha human brainwaves. It needs to resonate at this frequency for us to remain healthy. When this field becomes polluted it causes a number of problems for those living in the disturbed area. Some common signs of GS include chronic clutter, electrical faults, light bulbs frequently blowing, wasps and ants nests, ivy, nettles and twisted trees. There are a number of solutions for GS, including a variety of plug-in devices, such as the Raditech and the Helios. However, the most effective long-term cure is earth acupuncture, which works in exactly the same way as traditional acupuncture except you treat the meridians of the earth with large, wooden 'needles' rather than the meridians of the body with small, metal needles.

In this increasingly technological age I also check houses for microwave radiation and electromagnetic pollution with two different scientific field meters designed for this purpose. The EMFs around our homes represent a growing health hazard that we are only just beginning to comprehend. It is an area where my current research is firmly focused, as I believe there will be an explosion in health issues related to EMFs and digital technology as we begin to truly understand how these energies distort our natural magnetic fields.

To find out more on the Helios device, go to **www.mackail.com**. It also neutralises other electric magnetic pollution.

You will find more details on the Raditech at **www.integralnutrition.co.uk**. You can pay half the cost, try it for three months and if you don't think it's worked for you can get a full refund. I have the portable version – you can carry it to whichever room you're in, and even have it on in the car to neutralise all the negative energies coming at you from the ever-increasing number of mobile phone transmitters.

RADIATION SHIELDING PAINT

If you're in decorating mode, it's claimed that one way to reduce exposure to external radiation is to paint your walls and ceilings with a radiation shielding paint, available from companies like Ecos Organic Paints (**www.ecospaints.com**). You could consider doing this if you live in a flat where there are loads of transmitters on the roof, but beware that this is incredibly expensive and still requires more paint over the top. Also there's the issue of windows – you can't paint those. That said, chronic sufferers do report positive results from using this paint.

MAGNATHERAPY

I write at length in *Imperfectly Natural Woman* about my belief in magnatherapy and I do believe that in addition to helping our own bodies at a cellular level, magnetic devices can reduce our energy use and boost our protection against radiation.

There are lots of companies now promoting magnetic products but I still recommend one of the market leaders, Ecoflow (**www.ecoflow.com**), as their products are based on the same principles as those of the magnetic therapy used in hospitals. I have worn a magnetic bracelet – a Bioflow – for several years now and though I couldn't guarantee that it keeps me well I'm sure as heck not going to take it off to find out! You can wear the tiny magnets in the form of a bracelet or as a pendant and the theory is that with the magnet loosely against your skin, as blood passes through the field it's subjected to a magnetic pulsing effect, which is said to help the body maintain its pH balance, by regulating the blood flow. Good conductivity in the cells is maintained and the body keeps up a good level of alkalinity, which is essential for good health.

Also from Ecoflow, I have a Biophone attached to my mobile. If you can't do without your cordless phone handsets, place one on the base station and on each handset if possible (they're approximately £30). In a trial carried out on people claiming problems with mobile phone use, the Biophone was found to reduce complaints by a good 42 per cent.

Also gaining in popularity is the Green 8, a mobile phone protective 'foil' that sits inside your mobile phone to help protect you from radiation. It costs approximately £25 from **www.sheerprevention.co.uk** and is especially popular with teenagers who don't necessarily want to be showing off their 'concern', as it's neatly hidden inside the casing of the mobile.

This is a very complex subject, and scientific communities are continuing to disagree in all areas. I suggest that you revert to your own instincts and ask yourself, 'Could there be a problem?' My view is that there definitely is, and that precaution is the sensible option.

If this area interests you, see the website of the aforementioned Roger Coghill of Roger Coghill Research Labs. **www.cogreslabs.co.uk** or read his excellent books *Electropollution: How to Protect Yourself Against It* and *Something in the Air: The Hazards of Electromagnetic Technologies, the Benefits of Magnetotherapy and Electromedicine.*

IONISERS

Even though I'm trying to discourage use of electrical items, I do believe ionisers are a worthwhile investment. You can get basic ones for as little as £30 in Boots. They were popular in the 1980s but in truth there's no reason for them to seem any less necessary now. In the case of ions, positive actually means negative. Confusing, isn't it? I can't claim even a GCSE in physics but I'm assured negative ions are formed when a molecule gains an electron (stop there, I can hear you cry!) but you know how invigorated you feel if you stand near a waterfall or on a mountain top, well that's partly because of the high levels of negative ions. The positive ions found in quantities around polluted atmospheres can cause fatigue. Ionisers are said to put back the healthy negatively charged ions into the air and reduce the levels of air pollution, bacteria and viruses.

You can get personal ionisers and ones for use in the car too. Recently I've taken to using an ioniser when I'm working at the computer alongside a salt lamp and a plant. I point it directly at myself while working and I swear I feel a difference. If like me you spend long hours staring at a computer screen, recognise that you'll be exposed to high levels of 'positively charged' ions.

You can also now buy battery-powered personal ionisers, which can help tremendously with allergies. Really interesting, but sadly much more expensive, is the world's first therapeutic ioniser, the Elanra Mark 2. It's often used by holistic therapists, as it has over 100 different settings to treat insomnia, addictions, electromagnetic pollution and allergies. I fear I may soon be breaking the 'no electrical items in the bedroom rule' (see page 136) if I can borrow one and set it to 'lose weight while you sleep'. It may not surprise you to know they're not cheap at around £395, but if you suffer from allergies and insomnia it could be a good investment.

For more information, discounted prices and a personal telephone consultation, go to www.integralnutrition.co.uk.

HUMIDITY

Over the years most of us have created for ourselves a very dry centrally heated environment, in which the low humidity means that we sometimes wake up with a sore throat and in which keeping house plants alive is tricky. Years ago when I lived in a very dry modern house I invested in an electrical humidifier and an air-conditioning system. Thankfully a few years on and I've woken up to the fact that plugging something in to counteract the effects of my heating system is expensive and not ideal; humidifiers and air-con systems have potential for bacterial growth and just aren't needed. I now use a bowl of water to increase the humidity and notice that when the central heating has been on for a while the water evaporates very quickly. I'm now conscious that an overheated home is not healthy: I keep the thermostat on low and turn off radiators in rooms that are not in use.

PLANTS CAN HELP

It's well documented that indoor plants are incredibly beneficial in improving the quality of the air we breathe. One plant for every piece of electronic equipment is recommended. Quite frankly, in my place that would mean more plants than in Kew Gardens, but I realise I need to get some more and keep them alive – dead, flaky ones won't cut it!

Feng shui experts recommend peace lilies as excellent for diffusing the effects of electro-pollution. They're the ones with rounded leaves

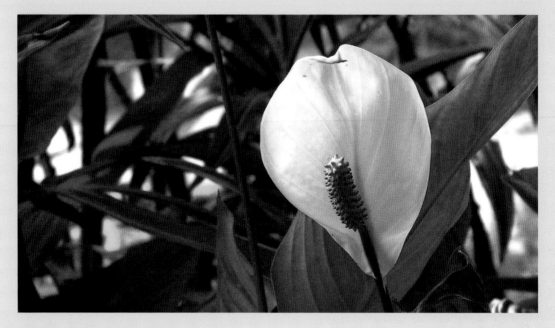

and white flowers. But avoid spiky cacti: I used to think these were good to have by a computer but now realise that they in fact simply make you feel 'spiky'– it's all a learning process! I've also changed my mind about having dried flowers and twigs around the house. Living energy is what you need to feel 'alive'.

Opt for easy-to-maintain plants such as spider plants, which I even managed to keep alive in student bedsits. One idea is to group plants together, as it makes it easier to water them and they seem to stay healthier.

Money plants are of course excellent for all kinds of reasons and actually pretty hardy. If you're interested in feng shui (see page 106), work out where your wealth area is and place a money plant right there.

ENERGISE YOUR HOME

So much of what I recommend is 'old style' and the next tip is too – and it costs nothing. It's simply to energise your home and improve the air quality in five minutes' flat. Open all the doors and windows – that's it! If you really want to shift some vibrant energy into the place, burn some incense. Make sure it's an aroma you like. I like the sandalwood one from **www.scentsofindia.co.uk** and it's eco-friendly, hand-made, Fairtrade and recyclable.

Do some of the 'space clearing' techniques recommended by Karen Kingston in *Clearing Sacred Space with Feng Shui*, such as clapping loudly in all the corners – yes, I know it sounds silly, but just try it; and if you've got one of those lovely Tibetan bells, ring it in every room. Finally put on some loud music – so long as you aren't going to upset the neighbours – and get cleaning!

Imperfectly natural home Q&A

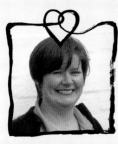

Leigh Smyth
Essentials for Equilibrium;
Holistic Health for
Animals and People

Describe your home.
Three-bedroom semi,
built in the 1950s by the
Forestry Commission to house the people
who worked in Kielder Forest.

Who lives here? I live here with my four
dogs and two cats.

**Have you attempted any eco DIY or
modifications for a greener home? E.g.
solar panels, eco paints, wind turbines etc.
Was it worth it financially?** I use a
Thermoflow device from Ecoflow, which is
a magnetic device that conditions fuel on
my central heating boiler. As soon as it was
applied, my radiators became hotter, so I
was able to turn down the thermostat. I
have oil-fuelled heating which is costly to
run, so any cost-saving is wonderful! I also
have a similar device fitted on my car to
help it use fuel more efficiently and
reduce emissions.

**How would your home rate for energy-
efficiency? What have you done to reduce
energy usage? When you buy new
appliances do you consider the energy-
efficiency?** My house is reasonably good;
it has cavity wall insulation and loft
insulation. I have a conservatory off my
living room, so when the sun shines I open
the doors into it and let the heat stream in
to the rest of the house. I do consider the
energy-efficiency ratings, yes.

**What cleaning/laundry/stain-removing
products do you use?** I use eco balls to
wash with, and my own blend of essential
oils as a fabric conditioner. I use a multi-
purpose detergent from a company called
Forever Living Products, which can be used
in the washing machine, on surfaces, floors,
carpets etc … it is very effective and claims
to be environmentally friendly and safe etc
… I use it on tough stains as a pre-wash
and for the dogs' beds in the washing
machine.

**If you have a garden what are your eco
tips?** Use a water butt. Make your own
compost. Mulch with crushed up pine
cones if you live near a pine forest. Leave an
area growing wild to encourage and
support insects and bird life. Also leave a
pile of logs/sticks to house insects.

What are your 'alternative' pet tips? Apply
the same principles to your pets as you do
to yourself: do not feed 'junk food', avoid
plastics in feed/water bowls etc …, use

natural products if you need to bathe the animal, use environmentally and animal friendly products. If you need pest repellents, use herbal ones (lavender is a favourite of cats and dogs. Grow a bush in your garden for them to roll in or leave a patch of lavender flowers on the ground somewhere so that they can roll in it if they need to repel pests.) Pests also dislike mint and other herbs, so have them available for your animals too (cats who roll in cat nip, which is a relative of mint, are naturally applying a pest repellent.)

Be aware that cleaning products may cause allergies in your pets, and that their sense of smell is very much stronger than ours (if you use something like a plug-in air freshener, for example, which is 'on' all of the time, imagine how your pets experience it, as their sense of smell is at least hundreds of times stronger than ours.) I could go on and on here, as this is my subject!!

What are your views on the possible dangers of electro 'smog'/wifi/emfs etc.? Have you take any protective measures?
I feel very strongly that we are polluting our environment too much with all of these extra currents and radiation. It does worry me, but I recognise that if I want the benefits of modern life, this is part of it. I try and minimise my exposure and risk by:

- Turning off my mobile phone most of the time unless I need it.

- I will never own a cordless (DECT) phone.

- I wear a Bioguard device from Bioflow.

- I take a supplement which has barley grass and wheat grass in, and also spirulina, as I believe that they will help my body fight the effects of this pollution. I keep myself as well as possible so that my immune system has the best chance of fighting anything that comes at it!!

What are your top three tips for a naturally healthy home?
- Get as much fresh clean air into the home as possible by opening windows every day.

- Have plenty of houseplants around to soak up pollution and negative energy.

- Clean your home with natural products and use ecloths as much as possible to avoid having to use cleaning chemicals at all. (also recycle old sheets and towels etc … as cleaning rags to use around the home instead of using kitchen roll for every little spill.)

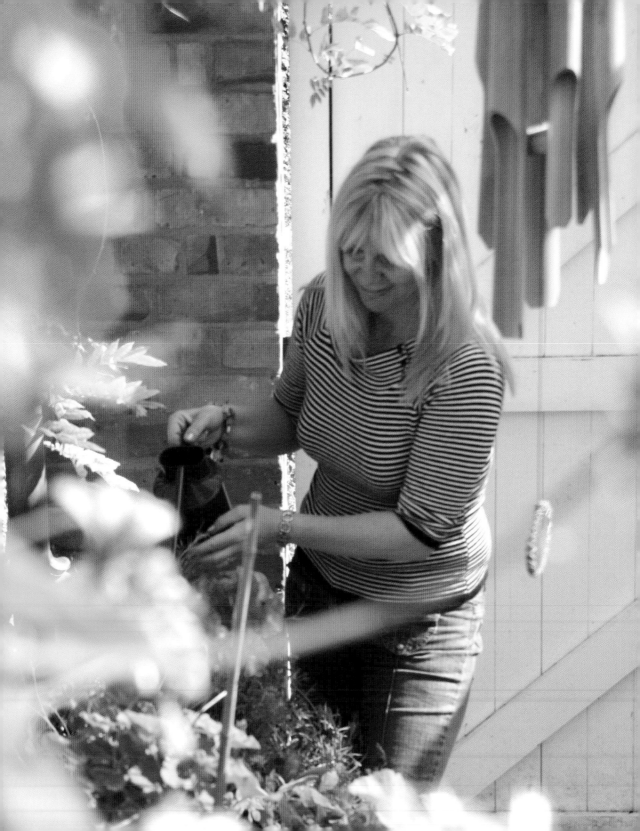

17 Let's go outside

'The best place to seek God is in a garden. You can dig for him there.'

George Bernard Shaw

Gardening is the new rock and roll … well, maybe after cooking. If you're lucky enough to have a garden, make the most of it. Gardens are healing and therapeutic, and of course incredibly useful, particularly if you can grow some fruit vegetables or herbs. I can't profess to be green when it comes to my fingers; though I love sitting in my garden, I have zero aptitude or patience for tending to the garden in any way. But I have many friends who find it the best form of relaxation (or indeed 'workout') that there is.

If you have illusions of grandeur à la Capability Brown, I warn you now that this chapter may be too simplistic for you. If, however, you love a nice garden but are just too busy, or you have merely a window box in your flat, I may have some ideas to inspire you. I'll pass on eco tips from my keen gardening friends and point you in the direction of some good websites. We spend billions on garden products every year, but in true Imperfectly Natural style, gardening really doesn't have to be an expensive pursuit.

Useful resources include **www.green gardener.co.uk** and **www.organic catalogue.com**; others are mentioned below.

ORGANIC – EASIER THAN YOU THINK

The best way to have a low-maintenance garden is to have an organic one. And it really is easier than you think. I managed to arrive there by default – well, laziness really. One of my mottoes is 'Intervention creates intervention' and I find if you 'leave alone', nature has a wonderful way of finding its own balance. Once you've passed on the chemical fertilisers, sprays and insecticides, and paid a bit of heed to companion planting, natural composting and encouraging a 'bio-balance' (see below), your own patch of green will pay you back with a loving natural smile. For more information on organic gardening, go to **www.gardenorganic.org.uk**.

You don't need to think big; in fact you don't even need a garden to go organic. When I lived in London, I nurtured two brilliant window boxes, and grew fantastic organic herbs and spices, practically all year round. If you do have a patch outside, and you're going organic from scratch, you have to allow a bit of time for things to adjust themselves, and you may have a year or so where things don't seem to be working. Gardens are sometimes called the 'great levellers' because they don't rush for anybody, but just stick with it, and I promise it'll pay off.

FINDING A BALANCE

Many of the problems associated with disease and pest control in commercial growing stem from the fact that growing huge areas of a single crop works against a natural ecological balance, and problem insects gain population advantages because of the absence of a food source for their natural predators. But most of us don't have 60 acres of corn growing in the back yard, and there's a great opportunity for us to avoid those problems by companion planting and mixing. Companion planting uses certain plants to deter the pests away from others. A good example is French marigolds planted next to tomato plants, which should deter aphids. To find which ones work best, go to **www.bbc.co.uk**. I dot different plants all over the place – herbs mixed with flowers, vegetables and salads mixed with ornamental plants. It's a bit of fun finding stuff sometimes, but I love the wild, haywire look of it all, and it makes the garden a place of leisure instead of another load of work to do. It's a real nature escape for me, which is what I want from a garden.

A recent survey found that many seeds were already dead when planted and many of the well-known brands didn't meet standards required, so be careful where you purchase your seeds from and ensure they're organically produced.

You can swap seeds with other gardeners at **www.seedypeople.co.uk** – a great way of getting rid of any surplus and trying out new varieties for the price of a postage stamp. You can also help the natural balance by encouraging wildlife into the garden, especially by providing feeding and nesting areas for birds. Just leave a small area completely wild for them to enjoy. For example, on average a pair of blue tits will collect up to 15,000 caterpillars in order to raise their young. My kids love those little natural wooden bird feeders – the kind you can often get in garden centres. I've occasionally bought some bird feed for the kids to leave out. If you love feeding the birds, consider their food miles too and opt for UK-grown seed crops from the Really Wild Bird Food Company (**www.streetendfeeds.co.uk**). If you want to really splash out for the birds, Natural Collection (**www.naturalcollection.com**) make a bird bath with a solar-powered water feature!

I'd also say leave your garden be, and don't attempt to make it too tidy. That old bit of

'Don't underestimate the therapeutic value of gardening. It's the one area where we can all use our nascent creative talents to make a truly satisfying work of art. Every individual, with thought, patience and a large portion of help from nature, has it in them to create their own private paradise: truly a thing of beauty and a joy for ever.'

Geoff Hamilton, gardener, author

rotting wood from a fallen tree, or pile of undisturbed rocks will be a habitat for all sorts of wildlife that will benefit your garden.

BIOLOGICAL CONTROL

One person who has applied a 'natural balance' approach to commercial growing is my good friend Mike from the fantastic Rocket Gardens. He manages to produce thousands of superb organic plants, completely avoiding the use of chemical pesticides and sprays, and instead introducing what he calls 'nice' insects to eat the 'naughty' ones that otherwise would be tucking into his plants. He says, 'Bio control is all about working with nature, not against it.'

Lacewings, ladybirds, predatory midges and parasitic wasps all help to control aphids. Predatory mites control whitefly, thrips and sciarid fly. You can actually buy these insects for your garden, and the plants that encourage them to thrive. Dedicated gardening books are full of information on native plants that attract helpful insects. Sometimes just choosing the right colours to mix in can introduce the right wildlife. More on this and bio control at **www.rocketgardens.co.uk**. Mike mixes flower plants such as nasturtium with vegetable plants such as cabbages to encourage good bugs such as parasitic wasps, hoverflies, lacewings and ladybirds. He says that companion planting can be an effective form of prevention against aphid infestation too.

Mike also says, 'Collect ladybirds whenever you see them and release them into your garden or greenhouse. Adult ladybirds eat greenfly and blackfly, but the growing larvae inflict the most damage on aphids. Pop them on your tomato and pepper plants and they will have a lovely time.' Natural Collection (**www.naturalcollection.com**) make a lovely silver birch ladybird house, where you can encourage them to thrive.

Oh, and a note on slugs ... Mike says, 'The best way to get rid of slugs is to pick them off after dark when they're out feeding. Don't just throw them over the hedge, as slugs are territorial and will return to your garden. If your compost heap is well away from your plants you can deposit them there. The good news is that if you clear them effectively, they shouldn't return for quite some time. Other "natural" techniques to deter slugs include beer traps, copper tape around pots and laying holly leaves around the edge of the garden.'

You can use biological control for slugs by buying parasitic nematodes. They're microscopic transparent worms which feed and multiply inside the slug. Dilute with water before use and ideally apply to moist compost or soil between April and September. Available from **www.gardening-naturally.com**.

There is a non-toxic slug killer based on ferrous phosphate (iron phosphate, which is an organic compound) plus a bait. Slugs and snails ingest the pellets and then crawl away to die, leaving no dead slugs or snails around and no unsightly slime. It's suitable for organic gardening. Available from **www.growingsuccess.org.uk**.

THE WEEDS

Remember that weeds are just plants growing in the wrong place. Some of the plants I really love to look at are what some would call 'weeds'. If you like them, just leave them.

Sadly there are no organic weed killers but if you're determined to kill them off but want to limit the damage, you can buy systemic weed killers that will kill just the weeds and not the surrounding plants; the chemicals are absorbed through the leaves of weeds, killing the plant as they travel through to the roots. One of the best ways to be weed-free, though, is to cover every available bit of soil with things you like, so that the weeds don't get a chance to grow. Alternatively if you don't like your garden to be too wild and crowded, use a good bark mulch – which you can buy from a garden centre – on any bare soil. Mulches go some way to keeping down weeds and also reduce evaporation, so helping to retain moisture in the soil. Spring is an ideal time to apply mulches but you can add them at any time as long as the soil is damp. Large containers can also be topped off with a mulch of bark or gravel. Gravel can be used as a mulch to keep the soil moist.

COMPOSTING

This is one of the 'musts' for organic gardening. As a nation we waste a staggering amount of food every year, and approximately eight million tons goes into rubbish bins. A whopping percentage of this could not only be composted but also used to generate power and even fuel if the infrastructure was in place. That aside, compost – i.e. green waste that has rotted down into a dark brown crumbly mixture – is a one-hit feed for your soil, full of nutrients, and it's free. For more on composting, see page 45.

A WORD ABOUT PEAT

From an environmental standpoint I always avoid buying this. Brilliant for your garden, but peat wetlands in the UK are ecological havens, and home to many rare organisms and species. Continued harvesting of the peat is endangering the delicate eco-balance in these areas, which can take hundreds of years to regenerate.

LAWNS

With the lawn, I don't mind a few weeds here and there. I'm also not big on over-manicured lawns and on that note it seems they aren't in fact terribly eco. I hadn't really thought about it until the recent water shortages, but lawns do require a lot of energy and fuel in mowing them, water for keeping them hydrated and chemicals to kill the weeds. One option is to abandon the idea of a lawn altogether but if you do want one it can be just as fun and lovely when you don't treat it as an outside carpet. Not cutting it so short by raising the lawnmower blades will help it retain moisture and stay greener. Obviously I'd say avoid using chemicals on your lawn as elsewhere in your

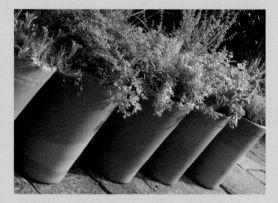

garden. Go the organic route and accept that a little clover, a few daisies and buttercups look great.

PATIOS

Patios were once the trend of the 1990s and are still a haven for most of us, where you can enjoy the benefits of a 'room in a garden', and as with your house, there are ways you can green it up. First of all, sorry, but there's just no alternative other than to ditch your patio heaters. There are still over two million of these in the UK, producing as much CO2 as 200,000 cars driving from Land's End to John O'Groats. That aside, it's got to be the most inefficient way there is to get warm. If you've got to have something out there as autumn rolls on, go for a chiminea (an oven for use outdoors), fuelled by dried-out wood or wood-burning briquettes. Kill two birds with one stone and cook your dinner on it at the same time.

Outdoor lighting is progressing in leaps and bounds, and self-contained solars are not only simple to install (you just poke them in the ground) but give you enough light to enjoy a few glasses of wine of a summer evening. These are now available everywhere.

If you're buying garden furniture, check to see if it is FSC certified, i.e. sourced from environmentally responsible and sustainable sources; some of the big store chains such as B&Q, Tesco and Asda actually do very well on this. And don't forget second-hand: not only is it eco, but a good measure of garden furniture quality is to see how it looks after a few years braving the elements.

If you're installing decking, avoid pressure-treated woods that contain arsenic. Maintenance wise, I like Osmo (**www.osmouk.com**), who make a good range of wood oils and treatments.

See also the excellent linseed paints from Holkham Hall in DIY stores.

I know we all love the Mediterranean look on our decks and patios, but I always try to give more than a nod here to good feng shui principles, by avoiding spiky plants. They look great in the catalogues, but you could be placing a load of 'dagger points' in your relationship corner, which absolutely won't be conducive to a happy, healthy home!

A citronella candle to ward off the peskies, and a glass of organic wine – and your patio will be almost a complete eco home in itself. How easy is that?

PONDS AND WATER

Ponds are a great way of creating a complete ecosystem in your garden, and the source of many a fascinating project for the kids. If you leave them alone, like the garden they'll find their own natural balance, and remain fairly maintenance free. Here's a snippet from my forum at **www.imperfectlynatural.com** between some friends discussing a few pond-related problems, a lovely little ode to how much fun they can be.

Hi Nikki,

As I said before, my view is that a pond is an evolving ecosystem. I try to not interfere with my pond too much, see how nature handles the situation.

I personally don't clean the sludge from my pond (wouldn't happen in nature sort of thing) but used different sorts of oxygenating plants over a period of maybe one to four years before the ones that are there now became established.

Strangely, the lilies that thrive the best I paid a pound for at a tiny nursery that was run from someone's house. I paid much more from aquatic centres for plants that did less well. My pond is now nine years old and still very much an ongoing project, but not a priority. It is very nice to sit out on a quiet evening and see the nature that happens all around and so close. We have so many types of birds, some bathing, some feeding, some just resting (we had a

kingfisher sat on a post for ten minutes once). Mind you we had a sparrowhawk doing what they do too. Nature is amazing.

If I can share what I have learned then feel free to ask.

Laurie

For more information on ponds, go to **www.gardenorganic.org.uk**. If you want to really make a splash with a natural swimming pool, see **www.naturalswimmingpools.com**.

SAVING WATER

There's lots we can do to save our precious plants from dying of thirst. It's always good to water in the morning or evening so as to let plants soak up the moisture before the hottest part of the day. If you water in the hot sun, water droplets on the leaves will act like little magnifying lenses, scorching the leaves. Also, as it looks as though hosepipe bans are likely for the foreseeable future, when you're investing in new plants or cuttings, choose ones that are naturally tolerant of dry conditions. Grey-leaved plants, such as lavenders, and santolina are fairly drought tolerant. Mulching (see page 148) is also a good way of conserving water in the soil.

'A pool is, for many of us in the West, a symbol not of affluence but of order, of control over the uncontrollable. A pool is water, made available and useful, and is, as such, infinitely soothing to the Western eye.' Joan Didion, author

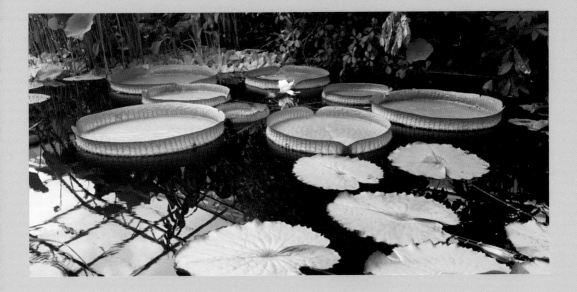

GREY WATER

When it comes to watering plants, my 'synthetic chemical-free' argument might fall down on its water saving butt, because I've been reliably informed that while putting used dishwater/laundry water – so-called grey water – on plants is a great idea, apparently it's not so great if you've been using some of the old-style stuff I've mention – for example bicarbonate of soda, borax, etc. don't react well with the soil and change its acidity level. Of course, you shouldn't use dishwater for edible crops, but it can be used for large shrubs. Make sure you let it cool off first, though.

RAINWATER

Rainwater is free from lime, and great for plants that don't like hard water. To save it you can now get water butts very cheaply and even make a garden feature of them with a pretty ceramic one.

British Eco (**www.britisheco.com**) sell a great range of products, from the Water Butt Jute Sack to my favourite, the simple wine barrel style, which looks great, especially in small gardens.

CAPILLARY MATTING

Capillary matting is great for standing pot plants on when you go away. It's a kind of felt, which sucks water from a reservoir, and into the roots at the bottom of the pots. It's used a lot in greenhouses.

For loads of information it's hard to beat the BBC website **www.bbc.co.uk/gardening**.

18 Pest control

The subject of pest control is a whole separate book in itself, but suffice it to say: avoid regular chemical treatments. There are lots of non-toxic techniques and products available, and simple environmental changes can easily reduce pest populations.

When was the last time you liberally sprayed around an insect spray to kill that pesky wasp, used flea powder on your cat or de-nitted your child with some highly toxic synthetic chemical shampoo? Many regular pest control products are laden with nasties that are not only hazardous to human health but also very un-eco. Household insect and fly sprays can contain pesticides such as permethrin and tetramethrin, straightforward biological poisons designed simply to kill living things, and even though they allegedly have low absorption properties in humans there have been reports showing permethrin, for example, occurring in breastmilk.

Eliminating a pest's food sources is often the best place to start. Many insects are attracted to something as simple as spilled sugary liquids or rubbish. Don't leave spills unattended. Many insects aren't too keen on basil, so keep a fresh pot in the kitchen – it smells great too. Structural openings and cracks should be repaired. A neighbour of mine once embarked on a rigorous poisoning routine to rid her roof space of rodents partying during the small hours, all to no avail. A few weeks later she blocked up their entrance with some wire mesh – end of problem. Now how old style is that?

On a cosmic note, consider the geopathic stress levels in your home (see page 137). Insects can be attracted to areas of geopathic stress, so if you have a constant problem with ants, and other pesky things like wasps, you'd do well to get any possible geopathic stress cleared. I know that at this point if you hadn't

'A man thinks he amounts to a great deal but to a flea or a mosquito a human being is merely something good to eat.' Don Marquis

considered it already you'll be wondering if I really shouldn't have been burnt at the stake for all my cranky ideas, but trust me there are those more cosmically creative than I! Karen Kingston in her fantastic book *Creating Sacred Space with Feng Shui* believes that all living things have an energy, and by using our own energies we can 'ask' them to leave (they might say no, though!).

MICE AND RATS

Let's start with mice, because they're quite frankly a devil to get rid of humanely. Mice basically look for food and shelter. Eliminating the latter is difficult, as they can squeeze into an opening the size of your little finger. The best way I've found is to simply remove their food source. Any little tasty scraps left around and one of them will find and tell all their mates. We had a serious problem with mice for a while, until we got more vigilant about cleaning up all the kids' half-eaten snacks from practically every room in the house.

The little critters even managed to gnaw away at my cloth nappies hanging over a drying rack. (They have an appetite for soft fabrics too.) I found some practical ways of getting rid of them, though. The little sonic devices from DIY stores work, until the mice get used to them, but I'd rather not have yet more plug-in things emitting some sort of 'wave' around the house. What about poison? Well, I wouldn't touch it with the proverbial barge pole. Aside

from the potentially terrifying consequences of your or someone else's young children getting hold of some of it, there's the fact that once the rodent has crawled off and died it will be excreting and decomposing, and some of the poisonous residues will end up if not under your floorboards, back in the food chain. I find the 'humane' traps a little odd. Taking a trek to the nearest field every morning holding a tiny wiggling box at arms' length so that you can give Jerry his freedom isn't really practical. Anyway, in the words of the great Basil Fawlty, 'They home.'

It's worth trying the non-toxic mice killer formulated from natural plant extracts which affects the digestive system of mice, available from **www.growingsuccess.org.uk**.

If you're desperate, the simple spring mousetrap is at least quick. Forget cheese: chocolate spread works well as a bait. A mean cat can earn his keep in the mouse control department too.

For rats, it's call in the cavalry, I'm afraid. I wish I knew a 'natural' way to be rid of them. Any tips greatly welcomed (other than of course owning or borrowing a 'ratter' dog).

WASPS

Avoid chemical sprays because they'll leave residues everywhere. I stick to old-fashioned ways of scaring them off. Last summer we used a citronella candle to ward off wasps, which seemed to work. You could also use a couple of drops of citronella or tea tree essential oil, and don't forget that an old-style low jam jar with a residue of jam or apple juice in it will catch them if you're hell-bent on drowning them. If it's a chronic problem, you could have a nest, and that's again a job for the cavalry.

MOTHS

Forget moth balls: they are frighteningly toxic – as most contain paradichlorbenzene and even the warning label cautions against 'prolonged breathing of vapour', so I'd say don't give them house room, especially if you have young children. Use lavender bags or cedarwood bars, from **www.clothworks.co.uk** or the Colibri natural moth repellent based on essential oils from **www.caraselledirect.com**.

If you do find that one of your old winter skirts has been moth-eaten, let it go. Nothing looks worse than a tiny hole and if you've left it for a long time without wearing it maybe it's time to get rid of it anyway (see page 108 [clutter]).

MOSQUITOES

Appearing more and more in the UK nowadays, mosquitoes love water, so clear puddles, and clean out drains, blocked gutters, bird baths,

kids' tyre swings, in fact anywhere you're likely to get stagnant water accumulating.

Change water in bird baths. If you keep fish, have some larvae-eating ones such as minnows and goldfish. Outside, yellow light bulbs as opposed to white ones are slightly less attractive to mosquitoes. There are some good natural repellents containing eucalyptus, citronella and even garlic. I find the Neem insect cream from **www.junglesale.com** works brilliantly as a repellent.

FLIES

Fly sprays like all insecticides contain toxins designed to kill living organisms. They are allegedly safe, as long as you don't inhale too much – an argument you could use for practically all the poisons on earth! I take the view that there's certainly less danger from a fly buzzing around your sitting room than from blasting a commercial fly spray about, and if you just open a window it'll probably buzz off. A more natural solution than fly spray in a kitchen is to hang up bunches of bay leaves or eucalyptus to repel flies. I remember an old aunt who used to fill little cloth bags with ground cloves, eucalyptus leaves and pennyroyal and hang them around in the summer.

If flies are a constant problem for you,

consider if there's something in the room that's attracting them – look for food spills, keep a tight lid on rubbish bins and keep open compost bins outside. Pyrethrum (a flower of the daisy family) planted near windows or doors will help repel flies and other insects. Their flower heads have been harvested for hundreds of years as a kind of natural insecticide, one of the few occasionally authorised for use in organic farming. It even occasionally turns up in fly sprays. Remember, though, that it's still a poison, and there have been reports of adverse effects in humans through overzealous use of pyrethrum in its more concentrated forms

ANTS

Also a nightmare to get rid of. I certainly wouldn't consider using commercial ant powder, but as a substitute you can use in the same way a mix of caster sugar and borax. Sprinkled cinnamon can work as a repellent too. Alternatively try applying tea tree oil or peppermint and simply blocking up the hole through which they are entering, if you can find it. If that doesn't detract them, then it may have to be a kettle of boiling salted water, if you can find their nest.

HEADLICE

I don't know if this exactly comes under the heading of pest control but they sure are a very annoying fact of living with children. For more on this subject, see *Imperfectly Natural Baby and Toddler*, but the bottom line is don't resort to scary chemical allegedly lice-beating shampoos: they are full of horrible chemicals and frequently don't work. Getting rid of nits is simple. It's all in the timing (based around the life cycle of the lice) and all you need is a fine nit comb and a bottle of conditioner. Check out **www.nits.net,** where they explain how to do it, and why conventional shampoos and the like don't work. Make sure you follow their instructions; otherwise you'll be de-lousing but will miss the tiny little babies just hatched. Preventatively it's a good idea to comb neem or tea tree oil through your child's hair if they're going to be in close contact with other children – or your own in fact, as adults aren't immune from the little blighters. Alternatively, use the new paraben-free version of BizNiz shampoo and conditioner from **www.lemonburst.co.uk** or the excellent Notnicetolice (**www.notnicetolice.co.uk**) range of shampoos.

Aaagh! I'm itching just writing this.

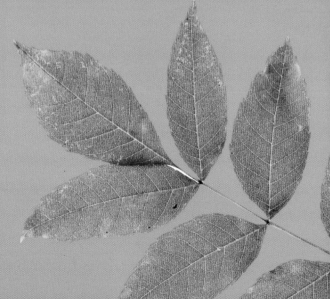

19 Natural pet healthcare

I don't have pets – somehow I've always seemed too busy or had too many children – but I have lots of neighbours and friends with animals. and often even if they haven't thought about organic food and complementary remedies for themselves they consider it for their pets, so thanks to my friend Alexandra Wood for this informative article.

When I first had my health food shop in 1995, customers would come in and select supplements and remedies for their pet, bring them to the counter and then look furtively around before whispering, 'It's actually for the dog.' This always amused me greatly and I often answered back with a big smile saying, 'That's OK, other customers have bought those for their dog as well.'

It's a booming industry, and recent research from a pet insurer found over 750,000 (14 per cent) of UK dog owners use alternative and complementary treatments, 30 per cent of which had been recommended to them by their vet, with 89 per cent saying that they would use these treatments again.

These are some of the remedies my customers bought: cod liver oil (the most popular) and garlic capsules; a lucky few were given royal jelly; aloe vera – both juice and gel (the gel being very popular for horse's legs); homeopathic and Bach flower remedies – excellent for animals frightened by the fireworks around Bonfire Night; along with essential oils; wheat bags – which when heated proved to be very beneficial for both new puppies needing the reassurance of a warm 'body' to lie next to and also those pets with joint and muscle problems; and Dog Oil … not heard of Dog Oil? It is an inexpensive, brilliant product originally used for racing dogs, excellent for joint and muscle problems.

Over the last 15 years, a lot of reputable companies have developed pet ranges to meet the growing demand from owners. From tinctures, essences and supplements, to creams, ointments and magnetic therapy products.

Essential oils were always a bit of a problem, as the dosage and toxicity varied with the size and type of animal – what would suit a dog would not necessarily suit a cat, even if they had the same ailment.

Homeopathy and acupuncture seem to be the most popular complementary/alternative

'Extraordinary creature! So close a friend, and yet so remote.'
Thomas Mann, novelist

treatments provided by vets. The British Association of Homeopathic Veterinary Surgeons (**www.bahvs.com**) and The Association of British Veterinary Acupuncturists (**www.abva.co.uk**) both have details on their websites of vets in your area that offer these treatments.

For joint problems, exercising in the water provides support and helps to relieve the pressure on weight-bearing joints, something which racehorse trainers and owners have made good use of for many years.

Pet massage is another area gaining popularity. My Reiki therapy teacher told me about her rescue cats and how they have benefited from the healing energy of Reiki (see **www.ukreikialliance.com**).

There's no placebo effect on animals, and my customers would often tell me of the improvements that alternative remedies and treatments had made to the lives and well-being of their animals. The enormously successful Bowen technique (see **www.thebowentechnique.com**) was actually first developed as a treatment for racehorses.

There are now many companies producing more natural and organic products from food to accessories, which will, no doubt, all help to make your dogs wag their tails with delight and your cats purr with pleasure, including: **www.dogoil.co.uk** for massage oil and virgin coconut oil; **www.naturalpetchoice.com** for hemp collars, toys and pet gifts; **www.junglesale.com** for neem pet care products, including a fantastic insect repellent. See also **www.essentialsforequilibrium.co.uk** for more on natural pet care.

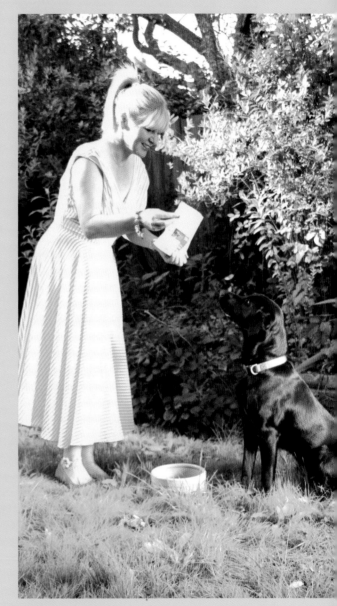

'Dogs come when they are called; cats take a message and get back to you.' Mary Bly

157

20 Money

BANKS AND BUILDING SOCIETIES

It's not so easy to check up on a day-to-day basis exactly what banks are up to, and I'm not certain we can expect banks to keep a track on every aspect of their customers' activities, so claims of 'green lending' for them is a difficult issue. Many a cynic would argue that banks have a financial duty to their shareholders to make money, and ethics largely don't come into it; that said, some definitely have a better 'green' track record than others. The Co-operative Bank (**www.co-operativebank.co.uk**) and Tridos Bank (**www.tridos.co.uk**) seem to fare pretty well.

Banks and building societies who advertise 'green' credentials may not necessarily be offering the best deals with regard to interest rates, costs and the like, so you may find yourself paying for the privilege of doing business with them. I think 100 per cent 'ethical finance' can be difficult to achieve and will be very personal; you have to consider not just savings and investments and your attitude to risk but borrowing wisely too. Financial products are confusing to understand at the best of times but when personal ethics come into it you may feel it's not worth the extra effort. However, there are some other simple financial choices you can make that can make

a difference (see below).

Ultimately, if more people start researching and choosing ethical investment, it will help convince banks and companies to be more accountable.

MONEY MATTERS

While we're all keen to 'reduce the waste' in other areas of our lives, let's not forget this with regard to our hard-earned money. The fantastic website **www.moneysavingexpert.com** will point you in the direction of the best deals for everything finance related, and there's also a thriving forum and newsletter to keep you abreast of the best deals, whether you're saving, investing or just running your daily finances.

FINANCIAL ADVICE

It can be worth taking independent financial advice, but opt for a company who are transparent in their dealings. For every financial product the consumer buys, independent financial advisers are usually given a huge commission, but financial advisers are just people like the rest of us, many having strong ethical convictions about the way they live and work. When I was looking to sort out my finances after selling a house, I went to Paul Fell of www.uksif.org. Paul is a great model for other IFAs to follow. He charges consultancy fees for his work but admits openly the amount of commission he receives from a company if you buy a product; what's more he offers a share of it back to the customer as an incentive (it usually works out that all his charges are covered and there's a tidy sum left over). In addition to that he donates a full 25 per cent of his turnover (not profits) to charities, which you yourself can partly nominate.

If you want to introduce some ethical credentials to your choice of financial institution, EIRIS (www.eiris.org) is a non-profit-making organisation that looks into companies' social, environmental and ethical policies and practices, including mortgage and insurance companies.

ETHICAL CREDIT CARDS

I like these. These are credit cards that give a small percentage of your spending to charities (their money, not yours) and there are loads of charities that you can choose from for where their donation goes, including the NSPCC and Cancer Research. The website www.charitycard.co.uk has an up-to-date list of what's available.

INSURANCE

For car insurance and breakdown services, consider an organisation that campaigns for alternative methods of transport. Don't worry, they won't leave you stranded; they're realistic enough to know many of us still drive cars! Go to www.naturesave.co.uk.

CHARITABLE GIVING

Gift Aid is a UK government scheme under which charities sign up and then for donation to them by a taxpayer, they can claim back the tax. To you, the amount is the same but they get an increase of your donation. If your church, youth club or school PTA is a registered charity but not claiming Gift Aid, encourage them to sign up. If you have 'quoted' shares (those listed on the Stock Exchange, bonds or land) to donate to charity, you can claim income tax relief on those and no capital gains tax will be due from the charity on the gift.

DIFFERENT DEALINGS

I've been a big fan of Time Banks for ages. The idea is simple: people exchange their skills and trade, for example, an hour's gardening work for an hour's cake baking. Each member has an 'account', and points are credited and

'Money is like manure; it's not worth a thing unless it's spread around encouraging young things to grow.' Thornton Wilder

debited accordingly. A similar idea is a local babysitting circle. I've been a member of one for years and it works a treat. Taking this idea one step further, LETS schemes (Local Exchange Trading Schemes) are becoming increasingly popular. Each scheme has a directory that widens the scope of people listed in the community who can offer swaps. See www.letslinkuk.org and www.timebanks.co.uk.

In Devon last year I saw several shops displaying the 'Totnes pound accepted' signs. These are a kind of local currency that works like a loyalty card and keeps trade circulating within the community. At the time of going to print the customer could spend £9.50 and receive 10 Totnes pounds to spend in local shops and businesses signed up to the scheme, which not only encourages local trade but reduces food and trade miles. Totnes is one of a growing number of what are being called 'transition towns' in the UK (see page 177 'Eco-future'). The Totnes pound is an interesting idea, which sparked a heated debate between DH and me. I think it's an innovative idea that promotes local communities; he thinks it's biased and 'isolationist'. The jury's out, I suppose, but there are alternatives to everything, even money, as Totnes has shown.

PENSIONS

Pension funds will want to make money for you of course, but again ethics may not be top on their list of priorities. You are, though, entitled to know your fund's 'Statement of Investment Principles' (SIPs are defined as 'the extent (if at all) to which social, environmental or ethical considerations are taken into account in the selection, retention and realisation of investments' – you'll find a definition in the small print). The potential for a fund's SIP to be mere lip service seems quite big to me, and interestingly, Friends of the Earth (www.foe.co.uk) recently ran an extensive survey enquiring into the efficiency of pension fund managers in actually carrying out their SIPs, and it was surprising, or rather not surprising, how many funds either refused to answer or scored very low. On the other hand, you may be the first to complain if your pension fund doesn't perform well. The arms trade for example, ethics aside, may be a very sound financial investment on paper, and has been in fact invested in by many a fund including trades unions, hospitals and charities. When it comes to your money, it's really not so easy being green!

ECO DEATH

Well, it's 'part of life', after all, isn't it? But not one we're crazy about planning for.

Often the simpler greener funerals are the ones that have the most meaning. Eco coffins have become much more fashionable as more and more people appreciate the unsustainability of burying new wood in the ground or burning it in a crematorium. The problem is that many coffins are made from chipboard with wood veneers, which are usually sprayed with formaldehyde. During a cremation, a high percentage of this is released as toxic fumes. If cremation has been selected, you can get coffins that don't contain any substances that pollute when burnt. For burials, you can now get coffins made from simple unvarnished pine, cardboard or even bamboo. Go to www.ecoffins.co.uk.

You can also go really green with a kind of shroud or 'sleeping bag' called an Ecopod; see www.ecopod.co.uk.

The greenest option of all is to choose to be buried if possible in land that can be converted to natural woodland. Mintel has published some research that said that 64 per cent of people liked the idea of being buried in a woodland or meadow, but there are currently only about 200 natural burial grounds in the UK and many of these are privately owned.

See Association of Natural Burial Grounds. www.anbg.co.uk

Companies like Memorial Woodlands (www.memorialwoodlands.com) specialise in these personalised funerals and they plant hundreds of trees each year, which are protected in trust from future development. Rather than erect a tombstone, people are encouraged to select a tree and wildflowers instead to mark a grave.

One inspirational place is Green Fuse (www.greenfuse.co.uk) in Totnes, Devon, which some say is the holistic capital of the UK. They have managed to give death a different image – the shop front is as unlike any other funeral directors' I've ever seen – and they clearly incorporate sustainability and fair trade into their ideals.

MAKING A WILL

Incredible, isn't it, that most of us don't do it until we have children and even then only under duress? Apart from ensuring that your loved ones are catered for and your funeral preferences are respected, a will is a good way of supporting causes that you believe in. Many charities offer the services of a will-making solicitor if you agree that they will be a beneficiary. For more information, contact your favourite charities direct.

Also consider whether you wish your organs to be used after your death. More info at www.uktransplant.org.uk.

21 Transport

'Drive slow and enjoy the scenery – drive fast and join the scenery.'

Doug Horton

CARS

I can't profess to driving a 'green' car. I just chose something relatively cheap that could accommodate my excessively large family. When my last car finally died on us I did go through all the considerations. Hybrid (answer: couldn't find one that I could afford or a six-seater), should I convert the engine to LPG, should I invest in a bio fuel tank, etc.? But in truth I've stuck with good old diesel, and I assuage my guilt by limiting journeys and having basically a 'green' approach to driving, by which I mean I use the car for essential journeys and even then don't do the boy racer thing (in my dreams, laden down with four kids, buggies, et al!).

I've also registered with Liftshare (**www.liftshare.org**). Whether you need lifts or can offer them, you save money and reduce the number of vehicles on the roads.

Many cities and towns now have eco taxi firms such as Greentomatocars (**www.greentomatocars.org**) in London and Biotravel (**www.biotravel.co.uk**) in Cornwall.

You may have seen the amazing Eco-one green racing car that was prototyped by Warwick University. The tyres are made of potatoes and the brake pads from ground cashew shells. The body was created from hemp and rapeseed oil, and it runs on fuel made from fermented wheat and sugar beet. I remember having a laugh with Steve Wright and Tim Smith on Radio 2, surmising that at least if you ran out of fuel, you'd have plenty to eat. Maybe that is taking recycling a step too far, but the good news is that it's easy to turn almost any car into a slightly deeper shade of green.

Eco-check your car

It's not easy, I know, but try to check a few items. Simple maintenance can reduce your fuel consumption and increase efficiency. Dirty oil will hamper performance, so change it at least every 6,000 miles. Believe it or not, you can get a kind of eco oil, which is basically just old oil cleansed of impurities and recycled. Absolutely fine to use – after all, we do it to drinking water. Old spark plugs will hamper performance too. Blocked-up air filters can increase fuel consumption by 12 per cent, and also check your fan belt tension – if it's too tight your engine will be working unnecessarily hard. All these things will save you mpg (miles per gallon), so next time the car's in the garage, ask them to do a quick check on them. An hour of a mechanic's time could lower your old carbon bootprint, save you a fortune, and reduce the wear and tear on your car.

Drive green

The faster you accelerate and drive, the more fuel you use. A roof rack will increase fuel consumption by slowing you down aerodynamically, so do you really need one? Using air con can increase your fuel consumption by 15 per cent, as can simply just revving your engine. Check your tyre pressure too, as incorrect pressures will increase fuel use.

The company Ecoflow (**www.ecoflow.com**) believe that it's possible to magnetically condition fuel to be more efficient. Their Motoflow fits to the fuel pipe of a car and is said to significantly reduce fuel consumption, particularly on older vehicles, and one of their best-selling products is the Thermoflow, which straps on to the incoming fuel line and is said to help reduce energy consumption. They also offer a money-back guarantee if you find it's not at all cost-effective within six months.

Bio fuels

It may surprise you to know that way back in the 1890s, Rudolph Diesel designed his original engine with the use of vegetable oils in mind, so while we're proudly congratulating ourselves on the buzzword that is bio fuel we should remember that he thought of it first. Of course bio fuels aren't perfect either. I always remember Jeremy Clarkson of *Top Gear* fame saying that chip oil was fine – 'Sieve out the bits and it's excellent,' he said – even for a high-performance car, but by the same token he reckoned bio fuel would never really be a sustainable option, as the infrastructure just isn't in place. The sustainability issue is an important one too, since we've all read about the demand for fuel crops, which could lead to destruction of rainforests and impact on the palm oil industry. It would be devastating if fuel crop growth took the land needed for food production. Certainly there is a school of thought that says if we are going to use bio fuels we must use crops grown in the UK, and there should be strict environmental guidelines for farmers.

Look at a possibility for the future: Organic Power (**www.organic-power.co.uk**) is an eco company who have a process of using waste to produce a clean energy source – now you're talking.

New car?

If you're splashing out on a new car, note that some now have energy ratings, rather like kitchen appliances, and of course if you drive a hybrid car you will be exempt from congestion charging in some cities. Also, **www.vcacarfueldata.org.uk** is a great website that helps you ascertain the carbon footprint of hundreds of new models on the market.

Electric cars are improving all the time. It seems that the government is dead keen to encourage us to buy them, offering breaks like no road tax, free parking on meters and bays, and again no congestion charge in London. One wonders how they would make any money from us if we all got one. For me they are only suitable for specific situations, mostly short journeys and non-motorway travel. I'm sure one day they'll rival petrol cars, hopefully before the oil runs out! Hybrids run on petrol and electric, taking the best of both, the great advantage being that the batteries are charged up by the petrol engine, thus avoiding having to plug them in. This was a serious contender for me had I found one large enough for my entourage!

Cars that run on Compressed Natural Gas (CNG) or Liquefied Petroleum Gas (LPG) are becoming more popular, the latter producing cleaner emissions and on offer at most big filling stations now. Again you will often get a reduction in your road tax and be exempt from congestion charging.

The Greenfuel Company (**www.greenfuel.org.uk**) convert petrol cars to run on LPG fuel, creating a dual petrol and LPG fuel system.

For ethical car insurance, see page 159 [Money].

Life without cars

It goes without saying, wherever possible use public transport, walk or get on your bike, but yet again I'm imperfect. I'll do the first two, but in truth I'm terrified of cycling on the roads. A recent initiative in London actually provided people with a 'bike buddy' – someone to assess their ability and then accompany them

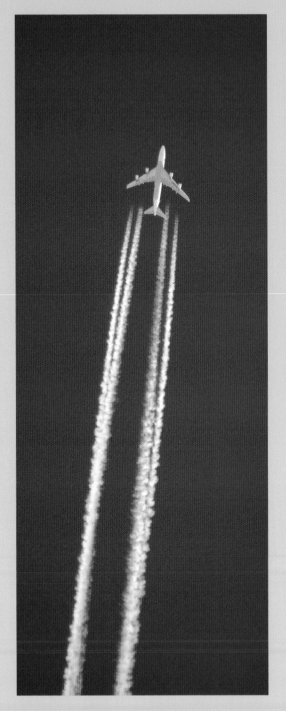

on a journey they often make. Fantastic idea. Don't be ashamed to admit you haven't cycled since you were a child, and get yourself a few proficiency classes. LifeCycle offers training and advice – see **www.lifecycleuk.org.uk**. Remember H. G. Wells once said, 'When I see an adult on a bicycle, I do not despair for the future of the human race.'

If you want to really have fun, check out **www.worldnakedbikeride.org**.

Worldnakedbikeride organise a day every year where they enlist the help of authorities of course and encourage people to cycle naked (body painting optional) to draw attention to how much fun and eco-friendly cycling can be.

Parents, look at **www.school-run.org**, a community website that aims to give children and parents increased opportunities to travel in a healthy and sustainable way, from finding lift sharing parents to accompanied walking.

CARBON OFFSETTING

I'm sure you've heard the joke – what's green and flies? An eco-hypocrite.

CO_2 seems to come in for a lot of stick at the moment. Yes, it's a contributor to global warming, but it certainly can't take all the blame. The recent trend for people to fly round the world but contribute to a carbon offsetting scheme has come under some fair criticism, I feel. Carbon offsetting is an exceedingly imperfect concept, rather like 'buying some forgiveness' for our sins. Some companies use the idea as a very tenuous way of appearing green, and the statistical evidence that one is actually offsetting is so open to interpretation that it's practically impossible to prove anything.

Carbon is an important issue, but we should perhaps take note that the UK accounts for less than three per cent of the world's CO2 emissions. Getting on my soapbox here for a minute, anything we achieve in reductions will have most world impact by setting an example rather than making a meaningful ecological difference. We must continue the good work in reducing our emissions, not by simply offsetting (which is basically continuing to pollute but assuaging our own guilt) but by aiming to reduce the amount of miles we travel where possible and encourage our governments to increase awareness in countries where pollution doesn't seem to be so high on the priority list.

Having said all of that, if you're going to be flying long haul, you may as well do your bit and contribute. Read more at **www.climatechange.org** and **www.carbonneutral.com**.

22 Imperfectly natural Christmas

I know there are people who choose to be on a beach on Christmas Day, and certainly if you're intent on long-haul travel, actually flying on 25 December will probably cost you less (in monetary terms), but in my view Christmastime ought to be about staying at home, or at least sharing the home with friends and family for a few hours or days. After the tender loving care your home has given you all year, reward it with your presence over the Christmas period.

If the whole idea of an all-singing, all-dancing 'commercial' Christmas makes you want to run for the hills, I sympathise. With four kids around I love Christmas at home, but I absolutely hate the expense of toys the kids will never play with, excess packaging and a mountain of food that we'll be hard pressed to get through. Fortunately, though, it is possible to have a green Christmas without being all bah humbug and wearing sackcloth instead of your regular party frock. There are loads of ways to make your home environment really festive while saving money and the planet at the same time.

CHRISTMAS CARDS

You probably noticed that you sent and received fewer Christmas cards, with many people choosing to send e-cards instead and donate the money saved to charity. Friends of the Earth (www.foe.co.uk) offer free e-cards from November.

Make sure you donate the cards that you do receive to a recycling scheme. The Woodland Trust has a scheme which recycles millions of cards, saving thousands of tons from landfill sites. You can donate them at certain high street stores and supermarkets.

If you want to make your own, consider using recycled paper. The Cutting Edge (www.eco-craft.co.uk) sell colourful blank cards and envelopes, all made from recycled paper.

CHRISTMAS TREES AND DECORATIONS

I have a huge artificial tree that I used to drag out every year until we moved to our present home, where it looks ridiculous, but if you've got one that looks good, by all means re-use it – just don't buy another artificial one! Being quite traditional, my house needed a real tree. I looked into buying a potted one that can continue to grow but found them to be very small. Next I considered a large one that could

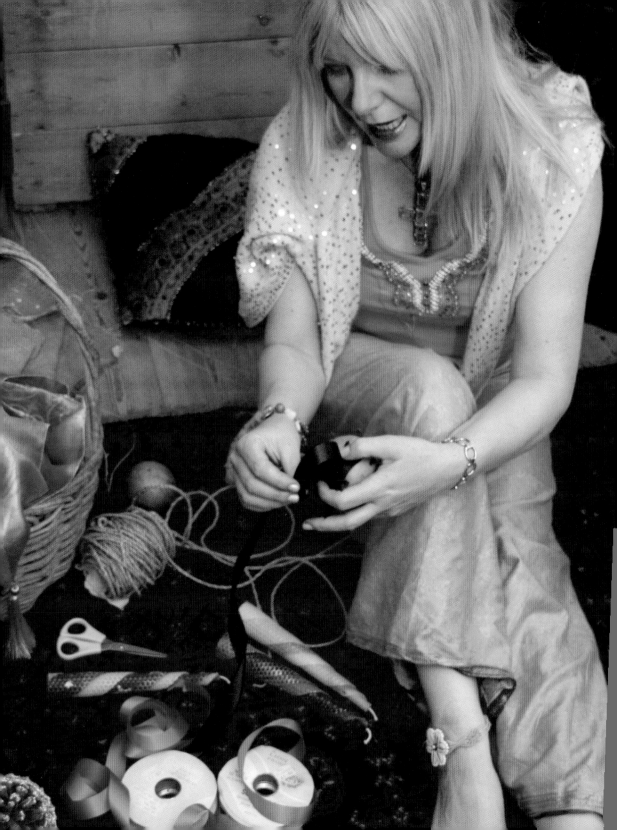

be recycled by the local garden centre, but in the end I decided to drape LED fairy lights over my huge plant instead. It worked fine. You can of course grow your own Christmas tree, but it will take a fair few years. Perhaps the best option if you want a tree is to buy one in a pot that can be transplanted into the garden such as a bay tree, which looks great all year. Holly is of course native to the UK and looks great.

A lovely idea for a gift, by the way, for any time of year is to send a small tree. Go to www.tree2mydoor.com who will send a lovely little tree – I have a gorgeous holly tree – and they'll personally inscribe a plaque to go with it.

You can also buy a friend a Tree Twist from www.treetwist.co.uk. This is a little piece of fabric that can be worn as a tie clip, a belt or a scarf, and for each one bought a tree is planted in the Caledonian Forest in Scotland.

If you do decide to buy a traditional fir tree,

SALT DOUGH DECORATIONS

Salt dough is a wonderful creative medium that lends itself perfectly to the making of Christmas decorations – frugal, easy and quick to prepare, it is also safe for children and has almost limitless possibilities, as far as your imagination will stretch.

300 g/10 oz fine salt
300 g/10 oz flour
200 ml/1.5 pints water
1 tablespoon vegetable oil (optional)

Mix the flour and the salt together in a large bowl. Make a well in the centre of the dry ingredients and pour in the water. It is possible that you may have to use a little less, or more water, so a gradual approach is best. Combine and knead until you have a smooth, non-sticky dough. Pop it into a plastic container to prevent the dough from drying.

To add colour to your creations, try adding spices such as cayenne pepper, turmeric, etc., cocoa powder or food colourings to the dough. Remember to knead the dough until the colour is uniform and smooth. Gloves are a very good idea to avoid multi-coloured hands.

Roll out the dough until it is about 1 cm thick and cut into shapes. You can use biscuit cutters in the shape of stars or Christmas trees, but leave a little hole at the top to pop string through. Lay them on a wire rack and leave to dry. Air drying is fine for small, thin objects. You can also leave them in the oven on a low heat until they are golden. Generally you should allow your creations to dry out for week before painting. You can seal your creations with a clear coat of varnish if you wish.

then check on **www.christmastree.org.uk** to find a British-grown one. Always make sure that you recycle it too. When you buy it, check that they offer a recycling facility, most garden centres do, or check with your local council for local recycling points.

At any time of the year if you love cut flowers think before you buy, as most are grown with a cocktail of pesticides and chemical sprays. Add to that the environmental impact of growing, packaging and transporting them. It's hip again to opt for dried flowers or silk ones (but don't let them gather dust), but better still gather your own fallen twigs. If you want a real treat, buy the luscious rich seasonal organic flowers from **www.tofc.co.uk**.

For tree decorations, I've never bought into the 'buying new ones every year' theory, but if you are feeling creative it's lovely to make your own little star-shaped ones from salt dough. This recipe (see left) comes from Amy Warburton at Brighter Blessings **www.brighter blessings.co.uk**.

Or you can get the kids to be creative with pine cones or bits of old coloured wool made into 'angels'.

To decorate the room I'd forget the tinsel and artificial bells completely and go for green. Literally deck the hall with boughs of holly. Collect ivy and other evergreens and just drape around liberally. Be careful with real mistletoe, though, if you have young children, as the berries are poisonous. Pampas grass looks good and wild clematis makes excellent natural

tinsel if you wind it into a wreath.

For that lovely festive fragrance, forget potpourri and just stick cloves into a big orange and hang it up with some red ribbon. Don't forget about it, though, as they do go off, which is not so fragrant!

If you've read the section on the importance of colour in your home (page 113), you'll know I'm a big fan of enhancing the mood and your own health and well-being by using cheap and cheerful artefacts, and decorative furnishings.

Comedian Jeff Green commented when he moved in with his girlfriend that he asked her if she regularly got power cuts because her home was festooned with candles, but the right candles can have great effect, and help give a homely ambience and a Christmassy feel. For more on buying and making candles, see page 171.

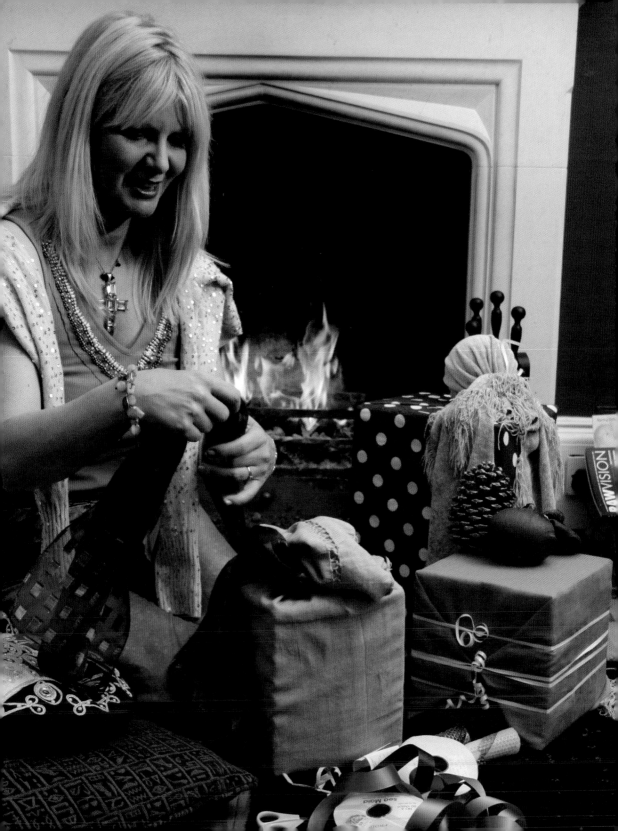

GIFTS

'One rose says more than the dozen'. Wendy Craig

For gifts I'd think personal and, wherever possible, home made. Yes, it really is the thought that counts and not the cost. One of the nicest gifts I received last year was a home-made gift of a little bag of pine cone firelighters. My friend Lynda – a very busy mum herself, which made it all the more impressive – had melted down some old beeswax candles by placing them in an old tin and then standing the tin in boiling water. Then she had poured the melted wax over the pine cones and added a few pretty star shapes, and around it went a sheet of cellophane and a green ribbon. It had pride of place by my fireplace all season. If you're any kind of domestic goddess, the possibilities are endless, including making little individual chocolates, tiny cakes or home-made fudge. Also much appreciated would be home-made natural soaps and lotions, and potions made with essential oils. If you're a novice, Neal's Yard (**www.nealsyardremedies.com**) will sell you all the base products you need. For high-quality organic essential oils go to **www.essentiallyoils.com**.

Candles are the new socks when it comes to presents. Beware, though, of petrochemical candles and opt for those made from natural beeswax. You can buy gorgeous candles from **www.brighterblessings.co.uk**.

You can make simple rolled candles with children. You'll need to buy wicking and wax sheets from a craft shop. Cut the wax sheets into 20 cm x 10 cm rectangles and lay them out with the small end towards you. Place the wicking along the 10 cm edge. It will need to overhang by about 3 cm, so trim it with scissors. Roll the wax tightly round the wicking until the entire sheet is rolled. You can decorate with glitter.

If you aren't the creative type and can't be doing with home-made gifts, give the gift of your time instead. Time is the one commodity many of us are short of, so if you have a skill or a service you can offer as a gift it could be hugely appreciated. For my birthday last year I received the most memorable gift of a voucher from a friend who offered to babysit my four kids for an evening – no mean feat!

A wonderful gift for any time of year for your partner or children is a 'voucher' book or book of promises. Get a petty cash voucher book from any stationer's and just write down your offer. So it could be: 'This voucher entitles the bearer to an undisturbed evening watching the football' or 'a full breakfast in bed'. To your friends you could offer your skills, so give them a voucher for three hours' gardening, or offer to cook a meal at their house for four people, or repair and alter their clothes if needlework is your skill – the possibilities are endless.

For children the vouchers can be as simple as 'a bike ride with Daddy' or 'an outing to the ice rink'. And of course this is a fantastic gift for children to give to their parents: they could offer 'a full tidy-up of my room', 'lots of hugs and kisses', etc.

You can of course give 'actual' vouchers too, such as a voucher for a therapeutic treatment, book tokens or theatre tickets.

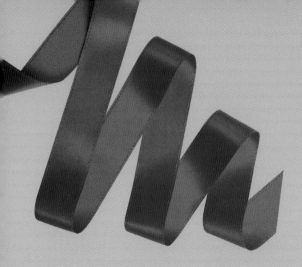

Many families now are setting a limit on the amount they spend on each person and agreeing to exchange gifts of only a fiver, for example. It's actually amazing what you can get for £5 if you include charity shops, and you can hold a bit of a competition as to who has found the most suitable perfect gift for another person that came in under the £5. Foodie gifts are usually appreciated too, so you could buy, for example, locally produced apple juice or honey, or a really nice olive oil in a beautiful bottle.

ETHICAL GIFTS

If all that 'make your own' just leaves you thinking, Oh stop it, let me just spend some money for once, then go for it. Just don't buy tat that will fall apart.

For kids' toys, look to sustainable wood toys, which are actually so much nicer to have around than brash plastic toys; and for art materials such as paints and crayons look to plant-based colours, which are wonderfully vibrant. For sustainable toys made from natural materials, go to www.ninnynoodlenoo.com and www.holtztoys. Try to avoid adding to the battery mountain too, and buy gadgets that are rechargeable or solar powered. There are some great solar toys for kids at www.selectsolar.co.uk. For more on sustainable toys, see page 95.

For gorgeous art materials and books, etc., go to www.myriadonline.co.uk. See also page 97 for more ideas of crafts with kids.

There are all manner of 'green gift' ideas now. Go to www.goodgifts.org and www.treehugger.com for some innovative ideas. You could buy the stationery lover a whole collection made from elephants poo (yes really) from www.natures-world.co.uk.

For the 'big kids' there are green gizmos and gadgets – see page 62 – and perhaps you can give gadget lover a power saver or an electricity-saving monitor, which in time will save them a small fortune and you all get to tick the 'eco box'. You'll find a wealth of products at:

www.ethicalsuperstore.com,
www.thegreenstoreonline.co.uk and
www.naturalcollection.com.

For lots of gifts made from sustainable materials or recycled products, see www.greenerstyle.co.uk.

GIFT WRAP

When wrapping gifts you really don't need to contribute to that huge excess paper mountain. (Apparently we throw out over 80 square kilometres of the stuff – enough to cover an area the size of Guernsey!) You can buy recycled gift wrap from the World Wildlife Fund www.wwf.org.uk.

There are lots of creative ways to wrap gifts, depending on their shape and size, from using remnants of old fabric tied with a fabric bow – hessian with red ribbon looks great – to making brown paper packages – (yes, tied up with string – 'a few of my favourite things'!). You can even use old magazine pages or newspaper – get the kids to give the paper a colour wash with some watercolour paint first, or just tie it with a big red ribbon. Try to make sure you've used some 'light news' pages, though, as it will take the edge off the gift if it's wrapped in details of a murder trial!

You can get a big piece of organic cotton

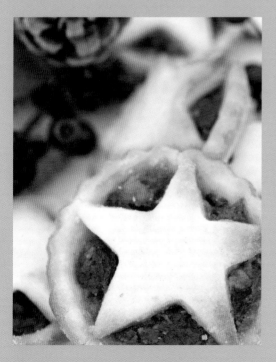

and make your own little drawstring gift bags or recycle old gift bags by adding new labels (made from recycled paper of course). If you want a gift box for something special, the Tiny Box Company (www.tinyboxco.com) have 100 per cent recycled boxes, which they'll personalise for you.

CHRISTMAS FOOD

Don't overshop. I mean it – we go mad, making shopping lists as if a famine was due, and fighting in the supermarket at 7 a.m over the best Brussel sprouts.

For Christmas dinner, don't panic. I'm not going to pretend to compete with Nigella here. I'd simply say if you're going to eat meat, make it organic and free range if your finances allow it. Know your turkey, or at least make sure your butcher does. For vegetarians I've never felt obliged to find a meat replacement for Christmas dinner, preferring instead to just have lots of really tasty roast veg, including some roasted sweet potato, butternut squash and red cabbage. For some excellent yummy vegetarian recipes, go to www.vegsoc.co.uk.

To cut through the grease, just make your own fresh cranberry sauce.

Make sure your wine and beer is organic to avoid headaches and your chocolates high in cocoa solids.

As far as possible, try to have a locally sourced Christmas meal and simplify. You'll feel the richer for it.

23 Eco-future

WHAT OUR HOUSES WILL BE LIKE

At some not-too-distant point in the future many of the ideals in this book will be simply 'bog standard'. All new home builds will be eco builds and it will be the norm rather than the exception to have all the environmentally friendly mod cons from the drawing board stage.

It's thought the ideal eco home will have ground source heat pumps, a system of pipes that absorbs heat from the ground and then transfers it to the hot water and heating system. Underfloor heating will heat from below (we all know heat rises); homes will benefit from a CHP boiler (see page 177), and an electricity generator will pass back any energy that is wasted back into the house via a heat exchanger.

Solar panels on the roof will heat water and photovoltaic cells will generate more energy, which can be stored in batteries.

Where possible some homes of the future will have 'living roofs, turf on the roof to help in the fight against climate change'. They could be covered with vegetation, and in some instances provide a garden space for city dwellers too.

A mini wind turbine will generate more energy to add to the mains supply, and perhaps most interestingly, the house will have insulated walls and roofs, but there will be ventilation with heat recovery, so fans will be positioned in a top room or loft and extract stale air from inside and draw in fresh air. A heat exchanger will transfer the warmth from the stale air to the fresh.

Sounds scary? It's coming to a home near you very soon. Almost certainly if you haven't considered one yet you'll be thinking soon about a Smart Meter, which allows you to see how much energy you're using in real time. I know I would be encouraged to save energy if I could see how much money I was saving just by turning things off rather than leaving them on standby.

Of course, the eco home would have a rainwater harvesting system, so that rainwater would be collected and used for flushing toilets. Hopefully there would be an effective grey water system for collection and re-use of bath and shower water too.

There are already some excellent models of sustainable homes. One such is the Beddington Zero Energy Development (BedZED) in south London, the UK's largest carbon-neutral eco-community and the first of its kind in this country. It is a mixed-use, mixed-tenure development, built on reclaimed land, which incorporates innovative approaches to energy conservation and environmental

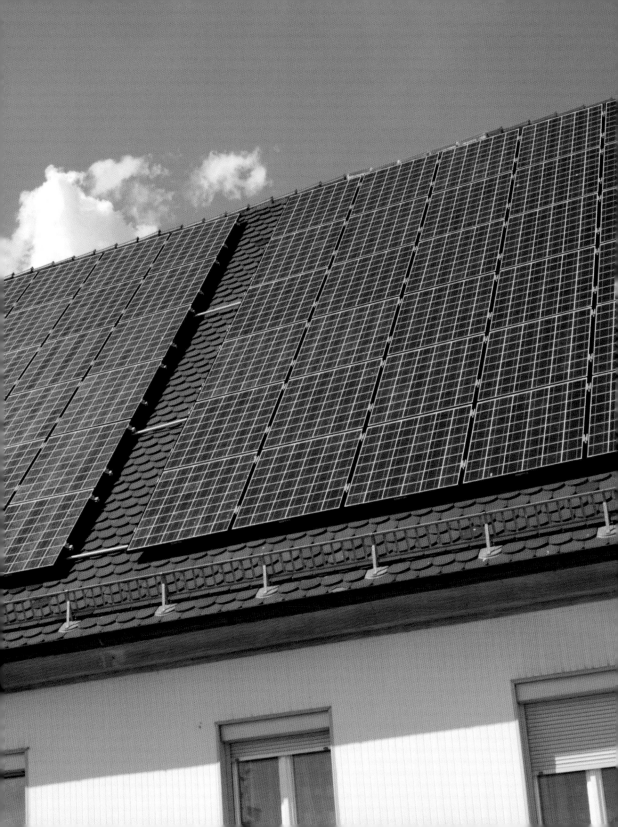

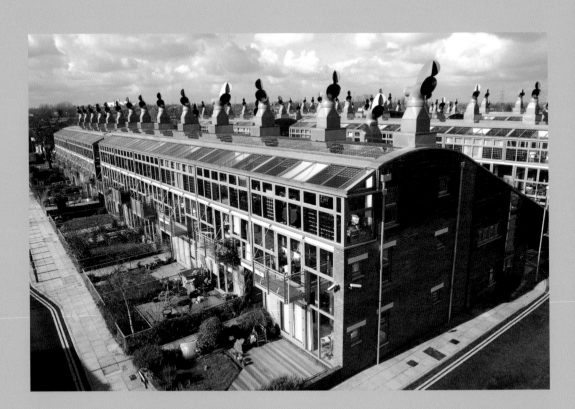

sustainability. The design concept was driven by the desire to create a net 'zero fossil energy development': that is, one that will produce at least as much energy from renewable sources as it consumes. BedZED is therefore a carbon-neutral development, because it makes no net addition of carbon dioxide to the atmosphere.

The design is to a very high standard and is used to enhance the environmental dimensions, with a strong emphasis on roof gardens, sunlight, the production of solar energy, the reduction of energy consumption and waste water recycling.

The buildings are constructed from thermally massive materials that store heat during warm conditions and release heat at cooler times. In addition, all buildings are enclosed in a 300 mm insulation jacket.

The houses are arranged in south-facing terraces to maximise heat gain from the sun. Each terrace is backed by north-facing offices, where minimal solar gain reduces the tendency to overheat and the need for energy-hungry air conditioning. Where possible, BedZED is built from natural, recycled or reclaimed materials. All the wood is FSC approved to ensure that it comes from a sustainable source.

Heat from the sun and heat generated by occupants and everyday activities such as cooking is sufficient to heat BedZED homes to a comfortable temperature; the need for space heating is therefore reduced.

BedZED receives power from a small-scale combined heat and power plant (CHP). Whereas in conventional energy generation, the heat that is produced as a by-product of generating electricity is lost, with CHP technology, this heat can be harnessed and put to use.

BedZED provides 82 residential homes of various sizes with a mixture of tenures. The project also includes buildings for commercial use, an exhibition centre, a children's nursery and a show flat so that visitors can see what it is like to live at BedZED.

A green transport plan promotes walking, cycling and use of public transport. A car pool for residents has been established. All these initiatives have helped to provide a strategic and integrated approach to transport issues.

For more on BedZED, see www.peabody.org.uk/bedzed.

Hardwood Homes (www.hardwoodhomes.co.uk) is another innovative company specialising in sustainable building design and construction, developing eco-friendly, green housing and commercial property development both in the UK and abroad.

Using a combination of sustainable materials, low-energy consumption heat and water systems, and environmentally friendly construction techniques, they aim to provide low-cost, desirable housing that will help reduce the environmental impact of our everyday living and create a sustainable environment for the future. They've got various projects in development.

TRANSITION TOWNS

A transition town is one that is exploring how to prepare for a carbon-constrained, energy-lean world. TTT is a community-led initiative working towards the creation of towns that use much less energy and resources than they presently consume and the design of more resilient, cleaner, more abundant and more pleasurable towns for the future.

The best example is Totnes in Devon, where sustainability is key. The use of the Totnes pound to reduce food and trade miles and keep money circulating in their community, which I mentioned on page 160, is one of the transition initiatives the town has used (At the time of going to print the number of transition towns across the UK is developing rapidly.)

For more information on transition towns, see www.transitiontowns.org.

There's lots of info too at the website of Climate Outreach and Information Network, www.coinet.org.uk.

Carbon neutral, sustainably built – these initiatives sound idyllic, don't they it? Sadly a BedZED home or the like is a million miles away from my draughty old Georgian town house. Of course there will always be old houses that can't be modified or adapted, but there are many other things that can be done towards a more sustainable and healthy future and I hope this book has provided a little food for thought.

Concluding hints and tips

So you've probably calculated your carbon footprint, done the maths as to whether you should consider a wind turbine or solar panels, convinced yourself that holidaying in Margate instead of the Maldives will be fine, and you've grown at least one slightly slug-eaten organic lettuce, but even with the best intentions, it's easy to take your eye off the ball.

Let's recap on the small changes that can make a big difference. Here's a summary of my tips (all described in more detail in the book) on how to live responsibly, do your bit for the planet and save your health in the process. Oh, and you'll have more money too.

THE WHOLE HOUSEHOLD

✓ Switch to a green energy supplier, and if you can get an energy monitor you're bound to be encouraged to economise.

✓ Fit some energy-saving light bulbs (but dispose of them responsibly). Most importantly, get into turning lights off.

✓ Check your house for EMFs.

✓ Make sure your home is well insulated and turn down the thermostat by one degree. If you have radiators, fit individual thermostats. Fit panels behind radiators to conserve heat, use old-style 'sausage dogs' (draught excluders) by doors and use heavy curtaining to retain heat lost through windows.

✓ Turn down your hot water temperature – 60°C is fine for taking baths etc. It's dangerous anyway to have scalding water coming from the taps.

✓ Sounds too obvious but save water by repairing dripping taps. They're bad from a feng shui point of view too.

✓ Fit a reverse osmosis water filter or use a jug filter, and don't buy bottled water.

✓ Recycle as much as you can. Nag your council to offer door collection.

✓ When re-decorating, use eco paints.

✓ When refurbishing, always seek out environmentally friendly or reclaimed materials.

✓ Fill your home with plants to purify the air.

✓ When treating woodworm and damp, avoid chemical treatments. Take advice from the Society for the Protection of Ancient Buildings (www.spab.org.uk).

✓ Reduce your paper mountain! Sign up to the Mail Preference Service to stop junk mail.

✓ Replace your cleaning equipment with eco chemical-free versions or go old style with the lemons and vinegar.

✓ Throw away, and never buy, chemical air fresheners.

✓ For special occasions such as Christmas, consider making your own gifts, re-use gift wrap and decorate your house with garden greenery.

KITCHEN/UTILITY ROOM

✓ Put kitchen waste into a compost crock and make regular trips to the compost bin. You'll be amazed how much you'll reduce your rubbish.

✓ Don't use kitchen roll to mop up spills; use washable cloths.

✓ Devise meal plans each week and buy only what you need. Make use of local suppliers and organic veg box delivery schemes. Avoid using too much processed foods and consider Fairtrade alternatives when buying all your goods.

✓ Decline excess packaging. Refuse plastic bags in shops, re-use the ones you have and get into the habit of carrying re-usable shopping bags with you.

✓ When your kitchen appliances start to get tired, see if they can be repaired; often fridges and freezers just need a serious defrost. When you do buy new, make sure you buy appliances with a high energy rating.

✓ Buy an eco kettle, or get into the habit of putting into your kettle only the amount of water you need before switching on.

✓ Use chemical-free laundry detergent, soapnuts or laundry balls, and set the machine to a lower temperature. Use vinegar and essential oils instead of fabric softener.

✓ Avoid tumble drying. Get an old-fashioned spin dryer instead, and/or hang out your washing on a line outdoors or an indoor pulley.

✓ When you must dry clean, use a Green Earth system.

✓ Use the dishwasher only on a full load and use eco tablets for detergent.

LOUNGE

✓ Clean carpets with 'natural' cleaners. Steam cleaners work well on stubborn stains: borrow or hire one occasionally.

✓ If you like fresh flowers, pick wild ones (be considerate) or buy organically grown flowers.

✓ When replacing flooring, consider natural options, such as jute, sisal or reclaimed wood.

✓ If you have an open fire – like imperfect old me – use eco logs or reclaimed wood.

STUDY/OFFICE

✔ Don't leave printers, mobile phones, etc. on permanent charge, and unplug your chargers.

✔ Consider going back to your old wired analogue phone system – you'll probably find a few corded phones in your loft!

✔ Use both sides of paper and use recycled paper where possible.

✔ Recycle envelopes and jiffy bags with recycled paper labels.

✔ Use peace lilies or even spider plants to neutralise the harmful effects of VDUs. It's thought that one small plant just 30 centimetres high can purify the air of a small room.

BATHROOM/TOILET

✔ Put a water saving device in the loo.

✔ Avoid toilet air fresheners and use a lifetime 'smell-buster'.

✔ Don't use bleach or chemicals to clean the loo, sinks or bath.

✔ Use recycled loo roll, as it biodegrades more easily.

✔ For the girls: avoid disposable sanitary protection and use a Mooncup or washable sanitary protection – cheaper, healthier and eco.

✔ When cleaning your teeth, always turn off the tap. Get a mug, camping style.

✔ Avoid regular harsh soaps and skincare products. Use natural beeswax soaps and 100 per cent natural skincare.

✔ Shower rather than bath, but if you shower for more than five minutes, you'll be wasting a scary amount of water. Bath with a friend!

BEDROOM

✓ Avoid electrical equipment, especially near your head when you sleep – no TVs or computers unless you have only a bedsit, in which case switch off at the wall at night. The only exception would be an ioniser if you suffer from insomnia.

✓ Open windows for ventilation and make sure you have heavy curtains that keep in the heat.

✓ Buy organic bed linen where possible and natural mattresses.

NURSERY/CHILDREN'S ROOM

✓ Use eco paints when redecorating and opt for plant-based colours. Consider sustainable wood for cots and children's beds. Choose organic bed linen and natural coir mattresses. Don't buy unnecessary equipment such as changing tables and furniture in the shape of toys. When relatives offer gifts, ask for high-quality natural toys. You can go second-hand for many children's items.

PATIO AND GARDEN

✓ Have a compost heap or recycled plastic compost bin and use it for kitchen waste; consider a wormery if space is tight.

✓ Never use pesticides or chemical fertilisers.

✓ Use natural pest repellents.

✓ Don't even think about patio heaters!

✓ Don't use disposable barbecues.

✓ Avoid peat-based compost products and use wormcast instead.

✓ Grow your own organic veg, cheating with bought-in plants if necessary.

✓ Even if you have no garden as such, herbs and small organic plants can be grown in pots.

✓ Collect rainwater for the garden in a water butt.

✓ When you replace garden furniture, consider recycled or at least sustainable wood.

LIFESTYLE

✓ Avoid buying gas-guzzling cars. Think before you use the car for short trips. Share lifts if possible. Sign up on **www.liftshare.org**.

✓ Don't throw away unwanted items: consider if they can be given away first. Buy recycled products instead of new whenever possible.

✓ Consider your wardrobe: buy fewer new clothes, however cheap, and repair and revamp old ones.

✓ For baby, consider re-usable nappies or at least eco disposables. Recycle baby clothes.

✓ Don't assuage your guilt by carbon offsetting – just choose a more eco option if possible (imperfections notwithstanding).

✓ Adopt an attitude of living more simply. You'll feel richer for it.

Directory

1. CLEANING

Green cleaning products
www.biodegradable.biz
www.clearspring.co.uk
www.daylesfordorganic.com
www.ecotopia.co.uk
www.ecover.com
www.faithinnature.co.uk
www.greenshop.co.uk
www.homescents.co.uk
www.junglesale.com
www.kinetic4health.co.uk
www.livingclean.co.uk
www.lemonburst.co.uk
www.naturalclean.co.uk
www.natural-house.co.uk
www.spiritofnature.co.uk

Cleaning tools
www.dri-pak.co.uk (bicarbonate of soda)
www.e-cloth.com
www.enjo.org.uk

Special cleaning
www.astonish.co.uk
www.auro.co.uk
www.perledeprovence.co.uk
www.shinypad.co.uk

Air fresheners
www.essentiallyoils.com
www.nealsyardremedies.co.uk
www.spieziaorganics.co.uk
www.vitalia-health.co.uk

2. LAUNDRY

Laundry balls
www.aquaball.com
www.ecoball.com
www.goholistic.co.uk

Soapnuts
www.ethicstrading.co.uk
www.inasoapnutshell.com
www.soapods.com

Dry cleaning
www.greenearth.co.uk

3. FOOD AND DRINK

Organic local produce
www.bigbarn.co.uk
www.farmersmarkets.net
www.seedsofhealth.co.uk
www.soilassociation.org

Organic food deliveries
www.abelandcole.com
www.ethicalfoods.co.uk
www.infinityfoods.co.uk

www.organicdeliverycompany.co.uk
www.purelyorganic.co.uk
www.riverfordorganics.co.uk
www.sheepdroveorganicfarm.co.uk

Superfoods – sprouts, herbs, etc.
www.bioforce.co.uk
www.creative-nature.co.uk
www.dreamacres.co.uk
www.livingfood.co.uk
www.steenbergs.co.uk

Wholefood shops
www.planetorganic.com
www.wholefoodsmarket.com

Vegetarian foods
www.buteisland.com
www.vegsoc.co.uk

Food in season
www.eattheseasons.co.uk

Grow your own
www.pfaf.org
www.rocketgardens.co.uk

Keeping chickens
www.omlet.co.uk

Sourcing fresh fish

www.fishonline.org

www.fish4ever.org

www.msc.org

Fish oil supplements

www.healthyandessential.co.uk

Slow food/foraging

www.inpraiseofslow.com

www.wildforestfoods.co.uk

www.wildmanwildfood.co.uk

Chocolate

www.divinechocolate.com

www.nourishme.info

www.rawintent.com

www.therawchocolatecompany.com

www.venturefoods.co.uk

Drinking water

www.ace-uk.co.uk

www.belu.org

www.deesidewater.co.uk

www.drydenaqua.co.uk

www.freshwatersystems.co.uk

Packaging

www.Ecolean.com

Beverages

www.cafedirect.co.uk

www.clipper-teas.com

www.ellaskitchen.co.uk

www.fairtrade.org.uk

www.festivalwines.co.uk

www.fortifiedcoffee.com

www.helfordcreek.co.uk

www.innocent.co.uk

www.juicemaster.com

www.realale.com

www.sunraysia.co.uk

www.vintageroots.co.uk

Cooking and cookware

www.1click2cook.co.uk

www.ethicalsuperstore.co.uk

www.lecreuset.com

www.pamperedchef.com

Composting

www.communitycompost.org

www.evengreener.com

www.greencone.com

www.lakeland.co.uk

www.wigglywigglers.com

4. RECYCLING

Shopping bags

www.bags2keep.co.uk

www.onyabags.co.uk

www.turtlebags.co.uk

www.zpm.com (trolley dolly)

Recycling and recycled goods

www.childrensscrapstore.co.uk

www.ebay.co.uk

www.freecycle.org

www.greenmetropolis.co.uk

www.junkk.com

www.mpsonline.org.uk

www.myskip.com

www.readitswapit.co.uk

www.recyclenow.co.uk

www.swapxchange.org

www.wasteonline.co.uk

www.which.co.uk

www.wrap.org.uk

New items made from recycled goods

www.greenerstyle.co.uk

www.junkystyling.co.uk

www.thegreenstoreonline.co.uk

Recycling initiatives

Computers for developing countries:

www.computer-aid.org

Computers for schools:

www.tfs.org.uk

Electronics: www.worktwice.com

Furniture: www.frn.org.uk

Mobile phones:

www.foneback.com

www.mobileamnesty.co.uk

Paint:

www.communityrepaint.org.uk

Tools: www.tfsr.org.uk

5. HEATING, LIGHTING AND ENERGY-SAVING

Home energy suppliers

www.downwithco2.co.uk

www.energysavingsecrets.co.uk

www.est.org.uk

www.foe.co.uk

www.good-energy.co.uk

www.greenhelpline.com

www.reuk.co.uk

www.resurgence.org

Solar

www.celticsolar.co.uk

www.selectsolar.co.uk

www.solarcentury.co.uk

www.the-green-apple.co.uk (solar toys)

Wind turbines

www.segen.co.uk

Heating and insulation

www.cvo.co.uk

www.ebc-ecofuel.co.uk

www.ecologicalbuildingsystems.co.uk

www.ecoutlet.co.uk

www.naturalcollection.com

www.recovery-insulation.co.uk

www.thecurtainexchange.co.uk

www.theshuttershop.co.uk

Power-saving gadgets

www.ecohamster.co.uk

www.ethical.superstore.com

www.greenwarehouse.co.uk

www.oneclickpower.com

6. HOUSEHOLD APPLIANCES

Energy efficiency

www.defra.gov.uk/environment

Ethical brands

www.gooshing.co.uk

www.healthy-house.co.uk

www.medivac.co.uk

www.miele.co.uk

7. NATURAL REMEDIES

www.avogel.co.uk

www.care2.com

www.cherryactive.co.uk

www.dreamacres.co.uk

www.eoco.org.uk

www.helios.com

www.hk4health.co.uk

www.indigoessences.com

www.junglesale.com

www.livingnature.co.uk

www.manukahoney.co.uk

www.mint-elabs.com (Z-gel)

www.revital.co.uk

www.sensitiveskincareco.com

www.supplementscompared.com

www.thebowentechnique.com

www.viridian.co.uk

Homeopathic remedies:

www.helios.com

www.homeopathy-soh.org

Medical herbalists:

www.nimh.org.uk

Menopause:

www.naturalhealthpractice.com

Nutrition advice:

www.bant.org.uk

www.integralnutrition.co.uk

Skincare

www.absolutelypure.co.uk

www.akamuti.co.uk

www.badgerbalm.co.uk

www.balmbalm.co.uk

www.coconoil.com

www.ecobath.co.uk

www.essential-care.co.uk

www.essentialspirit.co.uk

www.greenhands.co.uk

www.greenpeople.co.uk

www.highernature.co.uk

www.junglesale.com

www.kinetic4health.co.uk

www.lemonburst.co.uk

www.naturalspacompany.co.uk

www.naturalskincarecompany.com

www.naturaltoothbrush.com

www.nealsyardremedies.com

www.purenuffstuff.co.uk

www.rawgaia.com

www.sheerorganics.com

www.simplysoaps.com

www.spieziaorganics.com

www.tortuerouge.co.uk

www.trevarno.co.uk

www.trueaffinity.co.uk

Shower filter

www.sensitiveskincareco.com

8. PERSONAL CARE

Haircare

www.aubreyorganics.co.uk

www.lavera.co.uk

www.naturtint.co.uk

www.santecosmetics.co.uk

Deodorants

www.littlesatsuma.com

www.naturalcollection.com

www.pitrok.co.uk

Men's grooming

www.flintedge.com

www.greenpeople.com

www.nealsyardremedies.com

Make-up

www.drhauschka.com

www.inikacosmetics.com

www.lavera.co.uk

www.lemonburst.co.uk

www.lilylolo.co.uk

www.livingnature.co.uk

Fragrance

www.akamuti.co.uk

www.annemarieborlind.co.uk

www.florame.co.uk

Sanitary protection

www.drapersorganiccotton.co.uk

www.natracare.co.uk

www.mooncup.com

9. CHILDREN

www.babyscents.co.uk

www.cecebaby.co.uk

www.delicateskin.co.uk

www.greenface.co.uk

www.purepotions.co.uk

www.teamlollipop.com

www.thenappylady.com

www.trendykid.co.uk

Children's organic clothing

www.starchildshoes.co.uk

www.stella-james.co.uk

www.tattybumpkin.co.uk

www.uniform2.com

www.welovefrugi.com

Toys and crafts

www.brighterblessings.co.uk

www.ecochums.com

www.greatkidstoys.co.uk

www.holtztoys.co.uk

www.ninnynoodlenoo.com

www.littlehelper.co.uk

www.myriadonline.co.uk

10. CLOTHING, FURNITURE AND FABRICS

Clothes

www.beyondskin.co.uk

www.eco-age.com

www.eco-eco.co.uk

www.fashionpublic.com

www.gossypium.co.uk

www.greenshoes.co.uk

www.janknibbs.com

www.katherinehamnett.com

www.labourbehindthelabel.org

www.peopletree.co.uk

www.piccalilly.co.uk

www.sharkachakra.com

www.vegetarian-shoes.co.uk

Furnishings and fabrics

www.bluebanyan.co.uk

www.drapersorganic.co.uk

www.eco-label.com

www.foe.org

www.furnituretoday.co.uk

www.greenfibres.com

www.serenitysilk.co.uk

www.thecurtainexchange.net

www.woodnet.org.uk

11. ORGANISING AND CLUTTER CLEARING

www.firehorsefengshui.co.uk

www.flylady.com

www.mackail.co.uk

www.organisedhome.com

www.organisedmum.co.uk

12. LIGHTING AND COLOUR

www.apollo-health.co.uk

www.colourconsultancy.co.uk

www.litebook.com

www.philips.com

www.sad.co.uk

www.wholisticresearch.com

Himalayan salt

www.amazinghealth.co.uk

www.kudosrocksalt.co.uk

www.saltshack.co.uk

13. MOVING HOME

www.downshiftingweek.com

14. DIY AND MATERIALS

www.ecomerchant.co.uk

www.greenshop.co.uk

www.natural-building.co.uk

www.oldhousestore.co.uk

www.panelagency.co.uk

Eco paints

www.auro.co.uk

www.ecocentric.co.uk

www.ecospaints.com

www.greenbuildingstore.co.uk
www.villanatura.co.uk

Flooring
www.alternativeflooring.co.uk
www.forbo-flooring.co.uk
www.heuga.com
www.karndean.co.uk
www.naturalflooring.net
www.pandaflooring.co.uk
www.priorsrec.co.uk
www.urbaneliving.co.uk
www.zenflooring.co.uk

15. WATER
www.hippo-the-watersaver.co.uk

16. SOMETHING IN THE AIR
www.asphalia.co.uk
www.cogreslab.co.uk
www.healthy-house.co.uk
www.integralnutrition.co.uk
www.radon.co.uk
www.sitefinder.radio.gov.uk

Helios
www.mackail.com

Radiation shielding paint
www.ecospaints.com

Mobile phone protection
www.sheerprevention.co.uk

17. LET'S GO OUTSIDE
www.bbc.co.uk/gardening
www.gardening-naturally.com
www.gardenorganic.org.uk
www.greengardener.co.uk
www.growingsuccess.org.uk
www.organiccatalogue.com
www.seedypeople.co.uk
www.streetendfeeds.co.uk

Outdoor wood oils
www.gardenorganic.org.uk
www.osmouk.com

Water butts and rainwater harvesting
www.britisheco.com
www.thetankexchange.com

18. PEST CONTROL
www.caraselledirect.com
www.clothworks.co.uk
www.nits.net
www.notnicetolice.co.uk
www.thermolignum.com

19. NATURAL PET CARE
www.dogoil.co.uk
www.naturalpetchoice.com

Homeopathic veterinary surgeons
www.bahvs.com

Veterinary acupuncturists
www.abva.co.uk

20. MONEY
www.charitycard.co.uk
www.co-operativebank.co.uk
www.eiris.org
www.moneysavingexpert.com
www.tridos.co.uk
www.uksif.org

Insurance
www.naturesave.co.uk

Time banks
www.letslinkuk.org
www.timebanks.co.uk

Death
www.ecoffins.co.uk
www.ecopod.co.uk
www.greenfuse.co.uk
www.memorialwoodlands.com
www.uktransplant.org.uk

21. TRANSPORT
www.carbonneutral.com
www.climatechange.org
www.greenfuel.org.uk
www.liftshare.org
www.organic-power.co.uk
www.vcacarfueldata.org.uk
www.biotravel.co.uk
www.greentomatocars.com
www.lifecycleuk.org.uk
www.worldnakedbikeride.org

22. IMPERFECTLY NATURAL CHRISTMAS

www.brighterblessings.co.uk
www.christmastree.org.uk
www.eco-craft.co.uk
www.ethicalsuperstore.com
www.goodgifts.org
www.greenerstyle.co.uk
www.greengreenplanet.com
www.naturalcollection.com
www.natures-world.co.uk
www.thegreenstoreonline.co.uk
www.tinyboxcompany.co.uk
www.tofc.co.uk
www.treehugger.com
www.treetwist.co.uk
www.tree2mydoor.com

23. ECO-FUTURE: SUSTAINABLE GREEN BUILDING

www.hardwoodhomes.co.uk
www.peabody.org.uk/bedzed

Society for the protection of ancient buildings
www.spab.org.uk

MISCELLANEOUS

Eco holidays
www.bedruthanstepshotel.co.uk
www.ecovillagefindhorn.com
www.monktonwyldcourt.org
www.themagdalenproject.org.uk
www.trelowarren.com

Centre for sustainable future
www.csf.plymouth.ac.uk

Climate change
www.coinet.org.uk
www.transitiontowns.org

Green organisations
www.foe.co.uk
www.greenpeace.org.uk
www.unicef.org.uk
www.wen.org.uk
www.wwf-uk.org

Picture credits

John Moore: vii, viii, ix, x, 11, 14, 16, 22, 25, 26, 28, 31, 34, 42, 45, 47, 50, 62, 63, 68, 80, 82, 85, 96, 100, 107, 115, 116, 122, 128, 144, 157, 167, 170

Rex: 110, 121, 141, 151

Istockphoto: ii, 9, 21, 48, 78, 81, 133, 164, 169, 172, 173, 175

Mary Hennessy: 3, 88, 93, 149

Flickr: 57, 102

Corbis: 75

Zielonka Wohnen & Leben Gmbh, Germany: 18

BioRegional: 176

Photographic Stylist: Rosi Flood

Recommended Reading

Baird, Nicola, and Smith, Andrea, *Save Cash and Save the Planet*, published in association with Friends of the Earth, Collins, 2005.

Bonds, Lilian Verner, (Ra Bonevitz editor), *The Complete Book of Colour Healing*, Godsfield Press, 2000.

Bruce, Elaine, *Living Foods for Radiant Health*, Thorsons, 2003.

Butler, Daniel, and Crewe, Bel, *Urban Dreams, Rural Realities: In Pursuit of the Good Life*, Simon and Schuster, 1998.

Castro, Miranda, *The Complete Homeopathy Handbook*, St Martin's Press, 2003.

Cavitch, Susan Miller, *A Comprehensive Guide with Recipes, Techniques and Know-how*, Storey Books US, 1997.

Change the World for a Fiver: We Are What We Do, Short Books, 2004.

Chiazzari, Suzy, *Healing Home: Creating the Perfect Place to Live with Colour, Aroma, Light and Other Natural Elements*, Ebury Press, 2000.

Coghill, Roger, *Electropollution: How to Protect Yourself Against It*, Thorsons, 1990.

Coghill, Roger, *Something in the Air: The Hazards of Electromagnetic Technologies, the Benefits of Magnetotherapy and Electromedicine*, Coghill Research Laboratories, 1998.

Cuthbertson, Yvonne, *Success with Organic Vegetables*, The Guild of Master Craftsmen, 2006.

Hallows, Richard, *Diary of a Reluctant Green: Can you Save the Planet and Have a Life?*, White Ladder Press, 2007.

Hill, Ray, *Juice Therapy*, Nuhealth Books, 1997.

Honoré, Carl, *In Praise of Slow: How a Worldwide Movement is Challenging the Cult of Speed*, Orion, 2004.

Kenton, Lesley, *Raw Energy*, Vermilion, 2001.

Kingston, Karen, *Creating Sacred Space with Feng Shui*, Piatkus, 1996.

Lawrence, Felicity, *Not on the Label: What Really Goes into the Food on Your Plate*, Penguin, 2004.

Mabey, Richard, *Food for Free*, Collins, 2007.

Mackenzie, Aggie, and Woodburn, Kim, *How Clean is your House*, Michael Joseph, 2003.

Martin, Deborah L., *Natural Stain Removal Secrets*, Fair Winds Press, 2007.

Mindell, Earl, *The Vitamin Bible*, Arlington Books, 1999.

Norman, Jill (foreword), *Eating for Victory: Healthy Home Front Cooking on War Rations*, Michael O'Mara Books, 2007.

Norman, Jill (foreword), *Make Do and Mend: Keeping Family and Home Afloat on War Rations*, Michael O'Mara Books, 2007.

Onstad, Dianne, *Whole Foods Companion: A Guide for Adventurous Cook, Curious Shoppers, and Lovers of Natural Foods*, Chelsea Green Publishing Company, 2005.

Petrash, Carol, *Earthwise: Environmental Crafts and Activities with Young Children*, Floris Books, 1993.

Philips, Alasdair and Jean, *The Powerwatch Handbook: Simple Ways to Make You and Your Family Safer*, Piatkus, 2006.

Pilcher, Rosamunde, *The World of Rosamunde Pilcher*, Hodder and Stoughton, 1995.

Saunders, Kimberley, *Budget Meals: Eight Weeks of Delicious Dinner and Dessert Recipes*, Zodiac Publishing, 2007.

Saunders, Naomi, *Simplify Your Life: Downsize and De-stress*, Sheldon Press, 2006.

Statham, Bill, *The Chemical Maze: Your Guide to Food Additives and Cosmetic Ingredients*, Summersdale Books, 2006.

Thomas, Pat, *Cleaning yourself to death: How safe is your home?*, Newleaf, 2001.

Vale, Jason, *Keeping It Simple: Over 100 Delicious Juices and Smoothies*, Thorsons, 2007.

Vogel, Dr HCA, *The Nature Doctor*, Mainstream Publishing, 2003.

Waddington, Paul, *Shades of Green*, Eden Project Books, 2007.

Wren, R.C., *Potter's New Encyclopaedia of Botanical Drugs and Preparations*, Cosmo, 1985.

Wright, Angela, *The Beginner's Guide to Colour Psychology*, Colour Affects Ltd; 1998.

Index